PLANT-BASED KETO COOKBOOK

*Yummy, Easy and Healthy Recipes for Every Day.
4-Week Low-Carb and Whole Foods Plan
to Clean and Energize Your Body*

Jorge Moore & Melissa Drew

© Copyright 2019 - All rights reserved.

TABLE OF CONTENT

BOOK DESCRIPTION 5

INTRODUCTION 7

CHAPTER 1: Ketosis, Intermittent Fasting, Macros, and its Benefits 9

Starting A Ketogenic Diet 11

How Weight Loss Is Achieved in General? 13

Intermittent Fasting and Weight Loss Through a Caloric Deficit 15

CHAPTER 2: Foods to Avoid During Plant-Based Diet 17

Foods to Limit 17

Foods to Avoid 19

CHAPTER 3: Dealing with Cravings (What to Do When We Feel Cravings) 23

Tips And Tricks For Handling Carb Cravings. 26

Food to avoid during sugar detox period.................................. 28

CHAPTER 4: Foods to Eat During a Plant-Based Keto Diet 29

Fruits 29

Vegetables 31

Legumes 32

Whole Grains 33

CHAPTER 5: 30-day Meal Plan 35

Day 1 37

Day 2 41

Day 3 45

Day 4 49

Day 5 53

Day 6 57

Day 7 61

Day 8 65

Day 9 69

Day 10 73

Day 11 77

Day 12 81

Day 13 85

Day 14 89

Day 15 93

Day 16 97

Day 17 101

Day 18 105

Day 19 109

Day 20 113

Day 21 117

Day 22 121

Day 23 125

Day 24 129

Day 25 133

Day 26 137

Day 27 141

Day 28 145

Day 29 149

Day 30 153

CHAPTER 6: Maintaining a progress journal.................................... **157**

CONCLUSION **161**

BOOK DESCRIPTION

The book is conceptualized with the idea of offering you a comprehensive view of a plant-based diet and how it can benefit the body. You may find the shift sudden, especially if you are a die-hard fan of non-vegetarian items. But, you need not give up anything that you love. Eat everything in moderation.

As you start making the transition to a plant-based diet, you will find some remarkable changes within your body. You will have a better digestive system, and you can control chronic problems. All of these changes will make you happy in the long run. A plant-based diet alone can do wonders, but don't forget to exercise along with this diet to get the best results.

From the recipes and facts that are provided with them, it is proven that plant-based diet mainly consists of ingredients which are generally good for the health. Moreover, most of the nutritional benefits of the ingredients used in the recipes provide similar functionalities and benefits to our health. The most common and repeated benefits are lowering the risk of cancers and provide antioxidants to the body. This would further approve the fact that plant-based diet is an ideal diet for people who would like to transition from regular diet to plant-based as it contains almost similar nutrition with the regular diet plan.

INTRODUCTION

A fun way to get yourself used to this new lifestyle is to experiment with different recipes that sound good to you. You'll either realize that you like it and want to eat it again or maybe share it with the people around you if you live with others. Or maybe, instead, you'll be able to tell that it's something you don't like and wouldn't want to try again. Or maybe, it's just something you didn't like cooking. In that case, if you liked the dish but didn't like the work it took to prepare it, which happens to many people, that might lead you to a new restaurant that has the foods you can eat, and you might like how they prepare it. Once you begin experimenting and getting comfortable making the meals, it will become easier to adopt a new diet and find new foods that you like.

You can alter the recipes you already have and use on a daily basis too. If you eat meals with meat, make them vegetarian and then make them vegan before final making them ketogenic or Keto for short. You're still eating a meal that you already enjoy, it is just a different version of it. This can help you with your transition because it's just adapting things you're already used to. An example would be chili. Chili doesn't have to include meat at all, but if you really want it, try a meat substitute. Since beans aren't good for ketogenic because most of them are high in carbs, be sure to go through those carefully looking into the carb content and find a better option for that part of the diet as well. You could come up with an amazing recipe no one ever thought of before or you might be willing to try recipes that you wouldn't before this.

As you adapt to this lifestyle more and more, you should be able to stay on it much easier. Some good tips for maintaining your vegan lifestyle is if you like to eat out, it's like we said it can be difficult with your eating needs. So find out in advance where you can and can't go.

Have special food you can take with you when you leave your house. More and more places are trying to accommodate people's needs but some just don't have everything that you are able to eat because your diet can be a little bit restrictive. This is really going to help you keep yourself from being tempted by other's influence or choices or if a place you're at can't meet the needs of your diet. When you're out at social situations, it can be tempting to get out of your diet or eat foods you know you shouldn't. We have all been there. You can be at a dinner with a few friends and they want to share an appetizer and you think one won't hurt, or they want to drink so you figure one drink won't have too many carbs or something along those lines. A quick tip though; a lot of drinks do have carbs and on a ketogenic diet, it is really not recommended because you'll bust straight through your numbers. Some people even give in to the peer pressure because their friends get upset that someone is not eating like the rest of them. Ignore the peer pressure and do what you want to do. You don't have to answer to anyone but yourself.

Getting support will help you be able to stick to your diet as well. Having people around that love you and support you can be a very big help during this transition. Family can be a big help when you're making such a drastic change. If you are not able to be around encouraging people, then be sure to find motivation and encourage yourself. Too many diets come with negativity and people making fun of others for trying something different. If this is what happens to you, I am sorry because no one deserves that at all and it can be very painful for someone to have to go through. The best thing you can do is ignore the hate and keep a positive attitude and remember what you're doing this for. You're doing this for you, not them, and you don't need their negativity. Ignore it and brush it off and stick to what you really want. I know it can be difficult but just remember you don't need to keep that negativity around you and you are stronger than they are. You are the one that lives your life and you should be happy. Remember this and just keep pushing through. I recommend a reward for you as well. For instance, if you managed to stay a vegan ketogenic for a month, reward yourself with something you've been wanting, like a new pair of shoes or a movie that you've wanted to see. The act of giving yourself a reward will send a positive vibe to your brain that will reinforce your healthy habits and help you to want to keep going on your journey.

CHAPTER 1:

Ketosis, Intermittent Fasting, Macros, and its Benefits

The benefit of Ketogenic diet is that, it targets fat deposit in the most difficult parts of the body, most especially the abdominal region, thighs and the upper chest areas. Starving yourself may not help cut fat in the most difficult regions, even when you lose fat in such areas, they may return quickly, but this is not the case with Ketogenic diets. Losing weight around your mid-section and around vital organs is necessary in order to avoid serious fat-related diseases.

Ketogenic diets increase the amount of HDL cholesterols while reducing LDL cholesterol levels. Choosing the right type of unsaturated fats in your Ketogenic diet will help increase good cholesterols (HDL cholesterols), and these are healthy for the heart and general wellbeing. Ketogenic diets also help regulate blood sugar levels while reducing the risks of insulin intolerance. When carbs are broken down, they release sugar into the blood quickly and this increases blood sugar rapidly, a condition that triggers more supply of Insulin hormones, but when Ketogenic diets replace high carb diets, less sugar are released slowly into the body, a situation that can stabilize the secretion of Insulin hormones.

Ketogenic diet was coined out of the word "Ketosis", a process whereby the body breaks down more fat into fatty acids and ketones. The breakdown of more fats and ketones will provide sufficient energy sources for the body. Free fatty acids and ketones are simultaneously released in into the body during ketogenic breakdown, these are then made available for the body to burn as fuel.

Normally, the body relies on Glucose as the main source of energy, however, glucose is released when the body breaks down carbs, but the bad side of relying on glucose for energy is that, it can be readily stored as fat in fat cells, organs and tissues, when the energy is not used up. On the other hand, starving the body of glucose will force it to use stored fat in your organs as a source of fuel, even before they are stored for too long inside the body. With the burning of more ketones and fatty acids, there will be less glucose in the body to burn and the body will rapidly adjust to ketogenic phase of deriving energy.

You need to have it in mind that the body can only burn the source of energy present, therefore, constantly consuming ketogenic diet will make fats and proteins readily available as source of energy, as opposed to carbs. Ketogenic diets are effective in two ways, first, they create a net balance of energy in the body, and secondly, they rapidly fill you up (increase satiety), thus, you consume much less than necessary.

With Ketogenic diet, you have to avoid or limit your consumption of carbs to less than 5% of your daily dietary intake. Secondly, you need to avoid unhealthy carbs such as tubers, starches, sugar and other processes foods.

How does Ketogenic diet help you lose weight?

What your body is designed to eat will definitely affect whether you lose weight or not. The earliest humans often rely on what they get during hunting to survive, these include; edible foods, fish and meat, with little or no starch or carb, and that is one of the reasons why they stay slimmer and healthier. With the discovery of processed foods in the modern world (including pasta, white bread and sugary drinks), our bodies have been re-constructed to adjust to such unhealthy lifestyles.

One problem with most starch and sugar is that they can be converted into simple sugars that can be absorbed readily in the blood stream, and the effect of this is that there is a rapid increase in blood sugar level, a condition that triggers a sharp increase in the secretion of Insulin hormones, and this increases the risk of developing diseases such as diabetes type II through rapid weight gain and obesity.

One problem with carbs and sugars is that they increase your cravings, while Ketogenic diet helps you feel fuller quickly and reduce them. You can be at a dinner with a few friends and they want to share an appetizer and you think one won't hurt, or they want to drink so you figure one drink won't have too many carbs or something along those lines. A quick tip though; a lot of drinks do have carbs and on a ketogenic diet, it is really not recommended because you'll bust straight through your numbers. Some people even give in to the peer pressure because their friends get upset that someone is not eating like the rest of them. The early men consume more of ketogenic diets, and that is why they consume much less but get more energy for hunting expenditures. Ketogenic diets help lower your body's reliance on insulin hormones, and then makes it easier for the body to use up its fat reservoir as a source of energy.

You don't have to starve yourself to enjoy the benefits of Ketogenic diet, likewise, there is no need to start counting those calories.

Starting A Ketogenic Diet

Starting out on any new diet can be hard, but a ketogenic diet can be one of the hardest to start. This is because it is a sudden change to a completely different way of eating. Carbs are everywhere and we are programmed to eat as many as we can, so most of us have not had a carb-free day in our entire lives. For this reason, regardless of whether we are starting by reducing our carbs, or going cold turkey, the first few days need to be as easy as possible.

Make sure that you have got rid of all your high carb foods. Some people may do this by eating them all over a week leading up to the first day. Others may throw or give the food away to remove temptation. Either way, you need it gone before you start your diet, to remove all the foods that are likely to make you give up. For this reason, ask other people to keep their carby foods away as well, to prepare your own meals, and to refuse invitations to eat out for a while.

Make sure you have all the foods you will want to eat at home. Check out our recipes nearer the end of the book for an idea of what you will want to have. But the priority is a lot of leafy greens, low carb root vegetables, healthy fats, and lean proteins. If you can, try making meals in advance and freezing them in individual tuppers. And make sure to get some low carb, high fat, high protein snacks, like peanut butter, beef jerky, or boiled eggs. That way you can always have something quick to eat when you need it.

When starting out on a ketogenic diet, you will want to begin with foods you already like. Liver, kale, and almond butter are wonderful additions to a ketogenic diet, but eating things you don't like is not the best way to start a long-term diet. Instead, look through the recipe lists for recipes with foods you love, so that you can truly enjoy your diet.

Next, you will want to start on a morning, when you are not going to work. Stress makes us crave carbs more, and eating carbs is what starts the hunger cycle in the first place. You can be at a dinner with a few friends and they want to share an appetizer and you think one won't hurt, or they want to drink so you figure one drink won't have too many carbs or something along those lines. A quick tip though; a lot of drinks do have carbs and on a ketogenic diet, it is really not recommended because you'll bust straight through your numbers. Some people even give in to the peer pressure because their friends get upset that someone is not eating like the rest of them. So if we start with an empty stomach, running on ketones from the previous night, and we are going to have a relaxed day or two, we will be able to stick it out through the first few days. This massively improves our chances of success, as the first days are the hardest.

When you start a ketogenic diet, you will find many side effects. Most of them are harmless and just part of your body recovering from a lifetime on a high carb diet. Carb cravings are the most common symptom. We have already discussed why these happen, so it is important to remain calm and try and push through. In the next chapter we will offer some solutions for these hunger pangs, but remember that they are at their worst for only a few days, and after that they will be gone.

Indigestion can occur when you first start a ketogenic diet. This is due to a common mistake people make, assuming that this diet is low in all plants. That is not true. On this diet you will eat large amounts of high fibre, low carb plant foods, fatty fruits like avocado, and nuts and seeds. If you do not eat enough fibre you will find that your meals cause reflux, indigestion, and gut cramping. If you are eating plenty of plants but still suffering reflux, indigestion, and gut cramping, consider eliminating dairy from your diet. Sometimes following a ketogenic diet can make an underlying cow milk protein allergy come to the surface. You always would have had this allergy, but it would have been masked by other aspects of your diet.

Finally, if you suffer stomach cramps, diarrhoea, or oily, black stools, then you are eating too much fat. How is it possible to eat too much fat on a low carb, high fat diet? The same way it is possible to pour too much water into a glass. When we are following a ketogenic diet we are using fat as fuel. But we can only absorb so much fat in one go, and burn so much fat. You can be at a dinner with a few friends and they want to share an appetizer and you think one won't hurt, or they want to drink so you figure one drink won't have too many carbs or something along those lines. A quick tip though; a lot of drinks do have carbs and on a ketogenic diet, it is really not recommended because you'll bust straight through your numbers. Some people even give in to the peer pressure because their friends get upset that someone is not eating like the rest of them. When we eat more fat than we can absorb, our bodies just let it pass through us. This is largely harmless, but has the side effect of damaging our gut bacteria, one of the exact things we are trying to fix without diet. So if you notice these side effects, start reducing your fat intake until your stools return to normal.

Besides these symptoms, you should also experience a whole host of beneficial symptoms. Some of the most beneficial symptoms, like an improvement in metabolism, and weight loss, will take longer to happen. But others happen within days. You will find your appetite begins to come under your control. As your insulin spikes and crashes disappear, your body gets used to having a steady supply of energy. This means that rather than feeling hungry every single time your blood sugar drops, and snacking between meals, you are eating a healthy meal and going straight through to the next one without feeling hungry.

You will find that yeast infections and skin conditions improve, or even disappear entirely. This is because your candida is not being fed, so it has nothing to grow from. You can be at a dinner with a few friends and they want to share an appetizer and you think one won't hurt, or they want to drink so you figure one drink won't have too many carbs or something along those lines. A quick tip though; a lot of drinks do have carbs and on a ketogenic diet, it is really not recommended because you'll bust straight through your numbers. Some people even give in to the peer pressure because their friends get upset that someone is not eating like the rest of them. Candida causes many types of yeast infection, and several types of skin problem, being the root cause of most cases of dandruff, for starters. It also makes other conditions, like eczema, worse, by irritating the skin and growing under and around dead skin cells.

You will find your moods are more even. That "hangry" feeling you get when your blood sugar drops are not normal. It is your body responding to a lack of glucose, trying to get you to eat carbs. At first you may feel the carb-hungry anger more intensely than usual, but after a couple of days your body gets used to not having those constant spikes and crashes in blood sugar. No energy crashes mean no cravings, means no eating carbs, means no spikes, means no more crashes. It is vitally important to fight this cycle and restore order, even if you have no intention of following a ketogenic diet for life.

How Weight Loss Is Achieved in General?

Before we look at the best way that you can use intermittent fasting to help you reduce your body fat percentage, let's first quickly consider how weight loss generally works – think of this as the science behind effective and guaranteed weight loss.

When you eat something – regardless of what it is – it means you are putting calories into your body. Nutrients are broken down and absorbed by your body, while carbohydrates are broken down and then processed into glucose, which is then distributed through your body to provide cells with energy.

When excess glucose is present in your body, it will usually be stored as fat cells through a rather complicated process that we are not going to be discussing in detail here. As fat cells increase, you gain weight – ultimately leading to you becoming overweight and then slowly obese.

Now, on the other hand, when you are physically active – whether you are walking, dancing, or going hard on the treadmill at the gym – you are burning calories. Your body uses more glucose for energy, and when the reserves run out, the body starts looking toward stored fat cells in order to generate more energy. This energy then allows you to continue running on that treadmill or allows you to pick up the set of weights a few more times.

So, to sum this up – you eat, you gain calories; you exercise, you lose calories.

When the number of calories you eat surpasses the number of calories you lose, then you gain weight. Think of this within a 24-hour cycle. If you eat 2,000 calories, but only burn 1,000, then you gain weight to the value of those extra 1,000 calories that are left behind at the end of the day.

When you eat more calories than you burn, it means there is a caloric surplus. You are gaining weight and cannot lose weight with this strategy.

To lose weight, this entire equation needs to be in an opposite manner. You need to lose more calories than you burn. If you eat food that calculates to around 2,000 calories each day, you need to burn more than the 2,000 calories if you wish ever to see your fat go away and the number of the scale go down.

When your daily calorie intake is less than the number of calories you lose, then it means you have a caloric deficit – this is the ideal goal that you are striving toward when you are aiming to reduce your body weight.

Intermittent Fasting and Weight Loss Through a Caloric Deficit

With intermittent fasting, you still need to create a caloric deficit. I've seen some people think that simply because they are fasting, they will lose weight, regardless of the other factors in their life. This is not true.

No matter how beneficial fasting might be and a program that utilizes intermittent fasting, you will still need to take the science behind weight loss into account. If your caloric intake is more than how many calories you lose in a day, then you set the way for weight gain and not weight loss.

Intermittent fasting can make things a little easier, however. It has been found that people who follow an intermittent fasting program eventually experience improvements in their level of satiety. Their appetite is reduced, in other words. Since weight gain often lies within the fact that a person is unable to control their urges to eat inappropriate times, the reduced appetite will certainly be beneficial.

Additionally, because all meals of the day need to be squeezed into an eight-hour window with the particular intermittent fasting method that I am focusing on in this guide, it usually means that you will still feel somewhat full with your second meal after you had your first. When the time comes to have your third meal, the second meal will still be satisfying your appetite a little. You'll end up not wanting to overload your plate every chance you get – this means it becomes much, much easier than before to be in control of how many calories you will be consuming on a day-to-day basis.

Now, combine this with exercise. You won't even have to hit the gym too hard and may even be able to burn an adequate number of calories exercising at home if you are able to reduce the number of calories you consume by simply feeling full from the last meal when the time for the next meal comes.

CHAPTER 2:

Foods to Avoid During Plant-Based Diet

Now, we get to the fun part! If you still believe that a plant-based diet is going to be restrictive, be prepared to have your mind changed forever. The truth is, the plant-based diet includes a wide variety of foods that you get to enjoy. I know so many people who enjoy this diet and the benefits that go along with it; isn't it about time you join them?

To start off, we'll go over all of the incredible foods that you'll be enjoying. After that, we'll go in depth on the foods you should avoid on the plant-based diet. As mentioned earlier, there's a misconception that plant-based means no meat. That's wrong. You can still have the meat. However, after reading about the troubles it can cause to your health and our dear planet, you might want to limit it or even give it a miss. Once you have everything you need to know, be sure to read the next chapter where I've created an expandable grocery list for you, some delicious recipes and even a simple meal plan to help you get started. I want to give you as much help as possible so success is closer than you think in your plant-based journey.

Foods to Limit

In this next section, I will list off the foods you should still eat, but in sparing amounts. This means that even though they're allowed and do provide great health benefits, it doesn't mean you should eat them every day. That's because they also add a high amount of fat into your diet. This is especially crucial if you're looking to lose weight.

- Avocado

I said the same thing you're probably saying to yourself right now: Avocado is a fruit? Indeed, it is, but they are very different from your typical fruit. While most fruits are high in carbohydrate, avocado is low in carbs and acts more as an excellent source of healthy fats. The nutrients found in avocado include monounsaturated fat and oleic acid, both of which research has shown to be associated with better heart health and reduced inflammation.

- Nuts & Nut Butters

They are also commonly used as a healthy snack option. However, they do contain a relatively high fat content. The fat found in nuts include monounsaturated fat, omega-6, and omega-3 polyunsaturated fat. It should be noted that these fats are considered healthy, but you'll still want to consume them in moderation.

Examples: Peanut Butter, Tahini. Cashew Butter, Almond Butter, Walnuts, Pistachios, Pecans, Peanuts, Coconut, Cashews, Almonds.

- Seeds & Seed Butters

Just like nuts; seeds are a great snacking alternative. Seeds are extremely nutritious and are an excellent source of fiber. They could potentially help to lower your blood pressure, cholesterol levels, and blood sugar. However, it's true that there can be too much of a good thing. So, although seeds contain polyunsaturated fats and healthy monounsaturated fats, which are essentially good fats, they should still be limited. Examples: Sunflower Seeds, Sesame Seeds, Flaxseeds, Chia Seeds.

- Beverages

It should be noted that water is going to be the best beverage for you, but it is completely understandable if you don't want to just drink water for the rest of your life. This is why the following beverages are allowed, but should be limited to only a few times per week.

1. Fruit Juices
2. Unsweetened Plant Milk, eg. Soy Milk or Almond Milk
3. Processed Smoothies
4. Soy Yogurt
- Dried Fruits

Dried fruits are more processed compared to their whole or raw versions. If you do include dried fruits in your diet, you'll want to make sure that they are unsulfured. Some examples of dried fruits you could try include: Raisins, Medjool Dates, Currants, Cherries, Blueberries, Apricots, or Apples.

- Sweeteners

Adding a little sweetener is the secret ingredient to making yummy desserts or to satisfy your sweet tooth. However, you'll want to choose those that are minimally processed. I suggest looking for maple sugar, date sugar, or even cane sugar. On top of these options, you can always choose pure maple syrup. The goal is to make sure that you're getting real maple syrup and not something that is maple-flavored. These are very important differences you'll want to be conscious of when you start a plant-based diet.

- Condiments

When it comes to condiments, you'll need to be selective as well. While there are plenty of options on the market, you'll still want to select condiments that are going to be compliant with your new diet. Some of my favorites include Hot Sauce, Wasabi Paste, Vegan Worcestershire Sauce, Apple Cider Vinegar and Tomato Sauce. In the next chapter, you'll be gifted with a thorough grocery list to help you get started on your new diet!

Foods to Avoid

Here is where it might get tough for some of you. It is important to remember this phrase: "do not let the food control you." You are in control. You are the only person who can decide what goes into your body. The question is this, "do you want to fuel your body with nutrients or clog it up with unhealthy foods?" While it may take some work at first, you'll soon get used to it and naturally avoid these foods!

- Animal-based Foods

This is a given but remember that it isn't absolutely restricted! You SHOULD avoid them, but if you feel you absolutely need an animal protein, it is allowed in small portions. Some of the animal-based proteins you should avoid include fish, shellfish, game meats, chicken, turkey, pork, lamb, and beef. We have already gone over why meat might not be the best for your health, so how much of it you would allow in your diet is a decision you'll have to make for yourself.

- Eggs

This is another food that is tough for some people at the beginning. You'd be surprised to know that eggs are included in so many different types of foods. Whether it's your favorite bread or muffin, you'll want to avoid eggs (egg whites included). While it may be difficult in the beginning, it is absolutely possible to avoid them. So don't give in.

- Dairy

You'll want to avoid dairy while on the plant-based diet. This includes foods such as cream, yogurt, butter, cheese, and milk. You'll also need to be mindful of any food that contains a dairy product, or an ingredient made from a dairy product. As long as it is coming from an animal, like sheep, goats or cows, it should be avoided. Luckily, there're plenty of plant-based alternatives to keep you satisfied. Some examples are soymilk, cashew cheese, tofu yogurt, coconut whipped cream and frozen banana ice cream!

- Artificial & Refined Foods

Remember that this diet is all about consuming foods that are plant-based. From this point on, you will want to avoid foods that contain chemical additives such as preservatives, flavorings, or colorings. You'll also want to avoid any foods that have refined sugars or bleached flour. In the tips and tricks chapter, you'll be learning everything you need to know about reading a food label to help you avoid these ingredients. It can be tricky at first, but with some effort, you can say goodbye to artificial foods forever.

- Oils

If you are looking to lose weight, this is going to be a big factor for you! When you follow a plant-based diet, you'll be saying goodbye to any type of extracted oils. This includes fish oil, coconut oil, vegetable oil, and even olive oil! Don't worry, you'll soon find out once you get into the recipes section in the next chapter!

I understand this might be a lot to take in at once right now and I don't blame you if you feel a bit overwhelmed. However, I'm determined to provide you this information so as to give you a head start. By now, you should've understood the gist of it – whole foods are good; artificial foods are bad. The essential nutrients we need are found in both animals and plants, so why not choose the one that comes from plants?

One of the first questions I asked myself when I stumbled upon the plant-based diet was, "how is this diet going to be any different from the rest?" It is an important question as there're so many different diets on the market nowadays. Each diet claims to save your life, get rid of your disease and help you lose weight. At the end of the day, although not every diet is for everyone, you can never go wrong with being more conscious of what you eat.

The plant-based diet puts an emphasis on eating both fresh and whole ingredients. Basically, you are going to want to avoid food that has been highly processed. By eating minimally processed foods and increasing the plants in your diet, it will be effective in helping you to lose weight, improve your health, or both!

While there is no true definition to a plant-based diet, it is so much more than a diet. Most diets set you up for failure. If you're anything like me, you must have tried a handful of them already. Many individuals follow strict rules like cutting sugar, cutting carbs, or completely eliminating food groups that they love. Unfortunately, it's hard to do it this way because it's hard to just drop your bad habits. On the other hand, a plant-based diet doesn't have strict rules like these. Instead, it has basic principles that anyone can follow on their own time and pace. The best part is that it is inclusive, so you can make this lifestyle a family event!

Often times, a plant-based diet is confused with a vegan or vegetarian diet. The plant-based diet is the umbrella term where veganism and vegetarianism falls under. A plant-based diet is extremely versatile to help fit the needs of a variety of people. Yes, there is an emphasis on whole foods that have been minimally processed, but technically, animal products are still allowed on this diet, though they should be limited!

You'll be encouraged to learn how to enjoy new types of food such as nuts, seeds, legumes, whole grains, fruits, and vegetables. Later in the chapters of this book, you'll even be provided with a grocery list, meal plan, and the foods you should avoid and the foods you should enjoy. As I said, I'm setting you up for complete success here! When we do this together, we'll also be able to save our planet one healthy person at a time.

Of course, thinking about moving to this diet is going to be your first step. While it sounds like an excellent idea, often times it is difficult to know where to start.

CHAPTER 3:

Dealing with Cravings
(What to Do When We Feel Cravings)

Food has strong associations with memories, good times, and even love. There may be certain foods you've adored since childhood that are now out of reach because they are high in refined carbohydrates. These foods, strongly associated with comfort, tradition, and memories, may have an emotional pull that is difficult to resist.

Along with an emotional connection to food, there may be physical reasons for cravings, as well. If you've followed the Standard American Diet (SAD) most of your life, eating macronutrient ratios according to the USDA's food pyramid, then you've probably been eating a lot of refined carbohydrates. Foods high in refined carbohydrates can actually be addicting, according to a 2013 study from Boston Children's Hospital published in **Medscape Medical News**.

With that emotional connection, as well as a potential physical addiction to certain foods, it's understandable that cravings arise—even when you've made the choice to eliminate those foods from your life. The trick, then, becomes finding ways to manage these cravings while maintaining your healthy new lifestyle.

THE LOW-CARB LIFESTYLE

Choosing a low-carb lifestyle isn't a temporary solution to weight or health issues. Instead, it is a lifelong commitment to your health. Long-term success depends upon continued carbohydrate restriction. However, to realistically maintain the diet for a lifetime, you also need some sensible recipes that allow you to eat the foods you crave and still stay on plan.

Most diets provide tips and direction on how to succeed long-term and maintain weight loss and health gains. For example, the Atkins diet offers several phases that gradually ramp up healthy carb intake. By phase three and four, you move into pre-maintenance and maintenance phases, which allow you to make sensible choices for a lifetime of low-carbohydrate eating. Though you'll eat more carbs in these phases, you still won't be going hog-wild. You'll always need to restrict carbs on some level to maintain results.

By now, you probably have a host of recipes and meals that adhere to the plan's requirements. You know which foods fit your lifestyle and which are best avoided. Still, even with this knowledge and experience, cravings may lurk just around the corner.

Fortunately, there's no need to fall off the low-carb wagon to satisfy those cravings. You can give in a little by choosing modified versions of foods that are lower in carbs than their traditional counterparts. Of course, if you do eat these crave busters, the best way to balance this is to adjust carb counts throughout the rest of the day or week so carb levels stay close to those prescribed by your current eating plan and phase.

The recipes in this book remain very close to your low-carb plan allotments. While slightly higher in carbs than the typical low-carb foods you eat—some with as many as 5 grams of net carbs more than other foods—they aren't going to blow your entire carb budget. Instead of giving in to cravings with the "forbidden" versions of these foods, use these lower-carb versions to indulge, and adjust your remaining carb counts accordingly. Think of it as part of a winning strategy to maintain your healthy-living plan for the long term.

Your detox period will not be smooth, especially during the first days. They may even be worse than you'd expected. If this is your first time, you might be swayed to doubt that you're not doing it right. Doubts that maybe you're missing something. Maybe you ate something you shouldn't have eaten in the first place. You may then be tempted to abort the mission. "This looks like a mission impossible." But look, isn't it through the pain that you will gain? And just like any other road to success struggles and setbacks are involved? Same case here. Remember it can only get better. Your health is taking a step back before leaping forward. And you gonna love it and appreciate the sacrifice.

Just so you may be aware of the common side effects to experience during the detox period, here are some:

- Sporadic sleep, constipation and diarrhea, skin rashes/breakouts, cold-like symptoms, mucus drainage, headaches, low energy/exhaustion, bad breath, gas/bloating, and emotions resurfacing

But your reward is waiting for you. You will start experiencing the goodness of the cleansing even during the period and after. Talk about a clearer skin, better sleep, increased energy, increased sense of taste, fat loss, lower cholesterol, less depression, less bloating, regular bowel movements, and less sugar cravings. And there are many more benefits far much outdoing the sugar related problems.

You will crave that sugar. You will miss that food with refined sugar. The suggested foods herein are not as sweet as the sugars. But remember it is only for a short while and you will not to worry anymore when you see that cake. That honey in the kitchen looking at you like 'eat me please' because this craving will reduce and will have no force to make you have the temptation.

A times cooking might seem to be a time-consuming task. "I should probably grab some food from the shop, perhaps they say it's cooked well and has no sugars." That is not always the case. It is not an assurance either. Do you want to enjoy the full benefits out of the period? Then take time to cook for yourself. You might think that you have no time to cook but there's always time. Only if you plan well ahead. This guide has meal plans and recipes designed to accommodate two people. Probably you have a family member or a friend who needs the detox as you do. Or even more, huh. Working as a team is an added advantage. Encourage one another and together you'll reap the benefits of the period.

Even with this guide in place, you still should have a mindset for success. Sometimes due to unavoidable circumstances, you might miss following a part of the plan. What should you do? Set and discipline yourself to complete the detox period. Temptations are there, in plenty. Your friend's wedding is happening this weekend and you'd promised to attend. Obviously, there will be amazing sugary foods and beverages. "A small bite won't make much difference, will it?" Yes, it will. But there's a way around this temptations, besides the personal discipline. Take time and look for a period you will have no such plans to affect your detox. Plan ahead and you will have no problems.

Tips And Tricks For Handling Carb Cravings.

Carb cravings are one of the hardest parts of cutting your carb intake right back. We have already discussed why our bodies resist going low carb so aggressively, but that is of little comfort to someone who is going through the cravings themselves. Instead, here are some helpful ways of coping with the carb cravings until they naturally pass.

1: Sweeteners.

Although artificial sweeteners are hardly a health tonic, they can make for a very useful tool when controlling our carb cravings. Consider natural forms of sweeteners first, but most of them have a small amount of carbs, so if you will be using a lot, choose artificial ones.

Some people advise against using sweeteners, claiming that they will prolong the psychological addiction to carbs. However, although this is slightly true, it isn't the point. The physical addiction to carbs is far more intense than any psychological addiction, and if we go long enough without too many carbs, that addiction will break. After we have defeated the physical aspect of our addiction we can then consider cutting out sweeteners and fighting the psychological aspect. But until then, sweeteners are very useful.

2: Eat more protein.

Sometimes when we crave carbs we are just plain hungry. After so long eating too many carbs, all day every day, with every meal, our stomach rumbles and carbs are the first thing we try to get to eat. This means that we need to retrain our appetite signals to crave different foods, not just sugars and starches. And the first step to that is eating more protein. Eating protein fills our stomachs and triggers the release of hormones that make us feel satisfied. So if we need calories, protein should help.

3: Fill up on greens.

The annoying part of carb cravings, though, is that because they are so misdirected, they could be a craving for any vital nutrient. If eating protein doesn't satisfy you, then it might be that you need vitamins and minerals. A large green salad, or a low carb stir-fry or soup, will fill your stomach with fibre, and add vital nutrients to your diet. This can take longer to have an effect, so be patient. If it works and you feel better, increase your daily greens intake until you no longer feel cravings.

4: Drink some water.

And if protein and greens both fail, you might actually just be thirsty. When you rarely drink clean, simple water, your body doesn't know how to ask for it. Instead, it will fire up your appetite signals as soon as you get dehydrated. Get a glass of water and drink it quickly. Then get a second glass and sip it over half an hour. This rehydration might make your cravings go away.

5: Go for a walk.

Finally, if nothing hits the spot for your cravings, try and distract yourself. Mental activity can be hard in the middle of carb cravings, and idle distractions like watching television don't really take anything away from it. Instead, try and get moving. A walk around the block, or through some fields, can really take your mind away from cravings. And exercise, at least whilst you're doing it, will help you fight hunger. Just make sure to have a healthy meal ready for when you are done exercising.

6: Meditate.

Mindfulness is a great way of fighting cravings. You know, on a conscious level, that your cravings for carbs are not a vital need, that your body is misleading you, and that the cravings will go away. But your body, your primitive self, does not know that. It is thought that meditation is a way of communicating with your body and cooperating with each other. Some Buddhist monks can sit on solid ice blocks bare naked, or even slow their heart rates right down, without suffering harm, just by meditating and focusing on their bodies.

Food to avoid during sugar detox period

Vegetables

Tapioca, parsnips, boiled carrots, sweet potato, potatoes, French fries, pumpkin, corn

Grains and Refined Carbs

White rice, rye, wheat, brown rice, oats, wild rice, corn, sweet corn, long grain rice, barley, bread, cupcakes, couscous, candy, pasta, bagels, crackers, pizza, breadsticks, pita, croissants, brownies, pastries, English muffin, baguette, corn tortilla, doughnut, waffles, angel food cake, popcorn

Drinks

Sports drinks and almost all sodas and fruit juices

Sugar and snacks

Honey, syrup, candy bars, sugary snacks, sucrose, glucose, jelly beans

Fruits

Watermelon, banana, tangerines, dried dates, raisins

CHAPTER 4:

Foods to Eat During a
Plant-Based Keto Diet

One of the major benefits of the plant-based diet is that you can say goodbye to calorie counting! I mentioned earlier that the foods you'll be eating will be much more calorie-dense, meaning that you'll feel fuller more easily and for a longer time! You can say goodbye to counting calories and hello to actually enjoying your food! To begin, we will go over the foods that you can consume freely.

Fruits

While all fruits are allowed, it should be noted that not all fruits are created equal. Each fruit provides its own unique health benefits and coming right up, you will get my compilation of some of the healthiest fruits for your plant-based diet.

- Cranberries

Cranberries are unique fruits that are rich in vitamin K1, vitamin E, manganese, vitamin C, and copper! They also have a significant number of antioxidants that improve health significantly. Cranberries also contain A-type proanthocyanidins, which research has shown, to be a great help in preventing gum inflammation and urinary tract infections.

- Strawberries

Strawberries are among the most recommended fruits. It is also full of potassium, folate, manganese, and vitamin C. When compared to other fruits, strawberries are considered to have a low glycemic index, meaning they won't cause blood sugar spikes. A study published in the Anticancer Research journal has found that strawberries can actually prevent tumor growth.

- Mango

Mango is an excellent fruit to add to your fruit list, especially in the summertime! Mango has soluble fiber and provides vitamin C, which makes it anti-inflammatory. It also has strong antioxidants that lower the risk of diseases. In animal studies, it was found that the compounds in mangos could help protect against diabetes.

- Pomegranate

If you haven't had pomegranates before, you're missing out! Pomegranates are nutrient dense and have an excellent level of antioxidants to keep you healthy. In fact, a study published in the Journal of Agricultural and Food Chemistry has found that pomegranate juice has 3 times higher levels of antioxidants compared to red wine and green tea! On top of this, it's also full of different kinds of polyphenols, which reduces the chance of developing cancer.

- Apples

We have all heard it, an apple a day keeps the doctor away. As it turns out, there seems to be some truth to the saying! Apples are very nutritious and contain high amounts of vitamin K, potassium, vitamin C, and fiber! They also provide B vitamins. Research has shown that antioxidants found in apples can help promote heart health and may reduce the risk of Alzheimer's, cancer, and type 2 diabetes.

- Blueberries

Blueberries are most commonly known for their high levels of antioxidants, but they are also high in manganese, vitamin K, vitamin C and fiber! Jam-packed with all these nutrients, it's no wonder blueberries can help reduce the risk of certain chronic conditions including diabetes and heart disease.

- Pineapple

With just one cup of this delicious fruit, you receive all of the vitamin C you need for the day, plus a hefty amount of manganese too. Pineapple also has bromelain, which helps to digest proteins. In addition, studies have proven that pineapples can help fight and protect against cancer and tumor growth.

- Grapefruit

The list of fruits you can enjoy goes on and on, but I'll end off with grapefruit. Grapefruit is an excellent source of the vitamins and minerals. Research shows that grapefruit is associated with reduced cholesterol levels and may help prevent the forming of kidney stones.

Vegetables

On a plant-based diet, the bulk of what you'll be eating will be vegetables. Obviously, this does not come as a surprise. There are plenty of vegetables for you to enjoy, but the following are the real powerhouses that you'll want to include as often as possible into your diet.

- Brussels Sprouts

The truth is, it is all in the preparation! Brussels sprouts contain an antioxidant known as kaempferol. This specific antioxidant is linked to the prevention of any cell damage that is caused by oxidative stress, and is an important antioxidant to keep chronic diseases at bay. Additionally, brussels sprouts are an excellent source of potassium, manganese, folate, and vitamin C, A and K!

- Garlic

Rejoice all my garlic lovers! Garlic has many roots in our history as a medicinal plant. One of its main active compounds is allicin, and the research has shown that this compound helps to regulate blood sugar and promotes excellent heart health. It was also found in a study published in The American Journal of Clinical Nutrition that garlic is beneficial in lowering total blood cholesterol, LDL cholesterol, and triglycerides, all while increasing healthy HDL cholesterol.

- Broccoli

It also contains an abundant amount of potassium, manganese, and folate, which we need daily. Broccoli also contains sulforaphane, which has been found to have a protective effect against cancer. In one specific study, sulforaphane was successfully able to reduce the number and size of breast cancer cells while simultaneously blocking tumor growth.

- Carrots

In one cup of carrots, you'll receive 428% of your daily recommended vitamin A. Carrots also contain the antioxidant beta-carotene which is associated with cancer prevention. In fact, one study found that by eating one serving of carrots during a week could lower the risk of prostate cancer by 5%.

- Spinach

Of course, spinach is on the list! Spinach tops the charts as being one of the healthiest vegetables, and it isn't hard to understand why! Spinach is rich in iron, vitamin A, vitamin K, and is also packed with antioxidants. It also contains the compound called carotenoid, which the research has shown, can help individuals reduce their risk of cancer.

Legumes

While beans and legumes are more known for their fiber and B vitamins, they're also the main source of protein for your new, plant-based diet. Now, I will list some of the healthier ones you should make into staples, or when you're looking to switch out those animal proteins.

- Black Beans

Black beans might just become one of your new favorite foods. Not only are they packed with fiber and folate, they also offer 15.2 grams of protein in just one cup! These beans are beneficial as they have a lower glycemic index when compared to other foods with higher carbohydrates content. This means they can help control your blood sugar levels while being eaten as a staple. Scientists have even found evidence that black beans can help individuals manage their weight and type 2 diabetes.

- Kidney Beans

These beans are another food that is fairly common on a plant-based diet. Comparable to black beans, a cup of kidney beans contains an impressive 13.4 grams of protein. They are also high in fiber and are known to help slow down the absorption of sugar into the bloodstream. In the same study mentioned earlier, it was found that there is a connection between kidney beans and type 2 diabetes as well. On top of that, the fiber in kidney beans also helped to reduce the spike in blood sugar after finishing a meal.

- Peas

Peas are an excellent source of protein and fiber. They also have the ability to reduce insulin and blood sugar after a meal. What's more, you're not restricted to just plain peas anymore. Now, there is something called pea starch and it's also good for you. In fact, there is a study from the European Journal of Nutrition that discovered that pea starch could help you feel fuller for a longer amount of time.

- Lentils

In one cup of lentils, you'll get a whopping 17.9 grams of protein! The research has shown that eating lentils helps to reduce blood sugar and lower the risk of diabetes. Another study published in The American Journal of Clinical Nutrition has even shown that lentils can improve gut health by increasing your bowel function. When the stomach is emptied at a quicker rate, digestion increases and spikes in blood sugar is prevented.

- Chickpeas

The final source of protein that makes my list is chickpeas. They are often referred to as garbanzo beans and make an excellent source of fiber and protein. In one cup of chickpeas, you'll get 14.5 grams of protein. Specifically, chickpeas are great for reducing blood sugar levels and increasing sensitivity to insulin. It should also be noted that chickpeas can help improve bowel movement, by reducing the level of bad bacteria stuck in your intestines.

Whole Grains

As you switch to a plant-based diet, grains are going to become another staple in your household. Firstly, there are 3 types of whole grains – the bran, the germ, and the endosperm. Each one of these has its own nutrients, which are vital for your health. Whole grains are excellent as they are high in dietary fiber, B vitamins, selenium, phosphorus, manganese, magnesium, and iron!

- Quinoa

In South America, quinoa is a superfood! This is because this grain is packed with fiber, healthy fats, proteins and all the minerals and vitamins you need for a well-rounded diet. A study has shown that quinoa also contains the antioxidant kaempferol, (just like Brussels sprouts) and it helps in the prevention of certain types of cancers, heart disease and chronic inflammation.

- Brown Rice

For a majority of you, up until this point in your life, you've mostly been eating white rice. Yet, brown rice is the healthier alternative. This is because brown rice is a whole grain – it still has the bran and germ intact, which makes it richer in fiber, antioxidants, minerals, and vitamins.

Along with these benefits, brown rice also happens to be gluten-free, which makes it an excellent choice if you need to follow a gluten-free diet.

- Whole-grain Bread

On top of switching from white rice to brown rice, you'll also want to consider switching from white bread to whole-grain bread. There's a wide variety including whole-grain tortillas, bagels, rolls, and rye bread. Although it's a simple switch, you're actually adding more whole grains into your diet and this is extremely nutritious.

CHAPTER 5:

30-day Meal Plan

Below you will find 4 weeks' worth of meal plans and a shopping list to accompany it. The list will not have the amounts of the individual food you will need because that will depend on the number of servings. It also doesn't include basic things people normally have in their pantries such as oil, salt, pepper, and ground spices.

To use the meal plan you may use it exactly as is and write out the amount of each item you need or you may switch it up and make your own shopping list.

Day 1

Shopping list

- Chia seeds
- Non-dairy milk
- Natural nut butter of your choice
- Vanilla extract
- Maple syrup
- Tomatoes
- Cucumbers
- Onion
- Parsley
- Salt and pepper
- Virgin olive oil
- Balsamic vinegar
- Brown rice
- Lemon
- Vinegar
- Oregano

BREAKFAST RECIPE

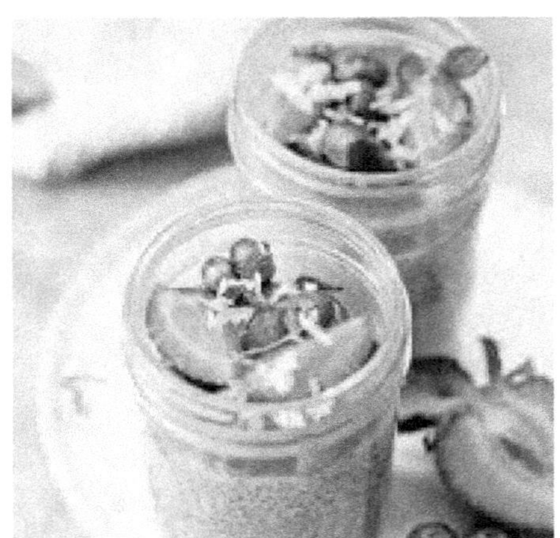

CHIA SEED PUDDING

Serves: 1
Calories: 379 per serving

Ingredients

- 2 tbsp chia seeds
- 1 ¼ cup non-dairy milk
- ½ tsp vanilla extract
- ½ tsp maple syrup

Directions

1. Mix together all the ingredients, cover. Put in refrigerator overnight.

2. By the morning the seeds will be hydrated and have the consistency of a pudding.

3. Pair with your favorite toppings. Fruit and oatmeal work well. Serve and enjoy!

LUNCH RECIPE

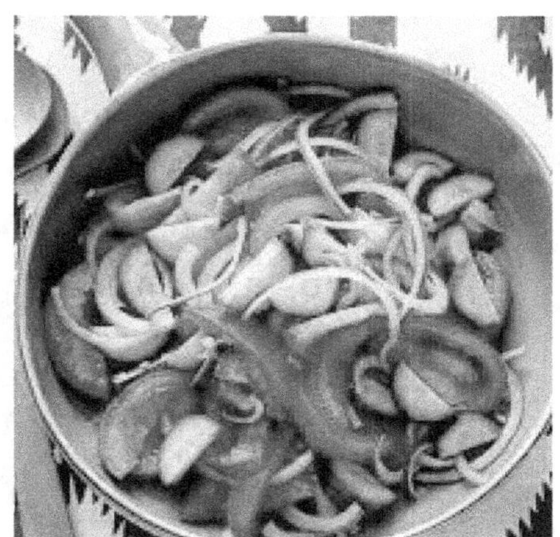

Tomato, Onion, and Cucumber Salad

Serves: 4
Calories: 84 per serving

Ingredients

- 4 medium tomatoes, cut into wedges
- 2 medium cucumbers, sliced
- ½ large onion (of your choice), thinly sliced
- 3 tbsp Parsley, chopped
- pinch of salt and pepper
- 1 tbsp extra virgin olive oil
- 2 tsp balsamic vinegar

Directions

1. Prepare vegetables and parsley; wash, dry, and cut.
2. Put in a large bowl and gently toss to mix.
3. Add salt, pepper, oil, and vinegar and gently toss again.
4. Plate, serve, and enjoy!

DINNER RECIPE

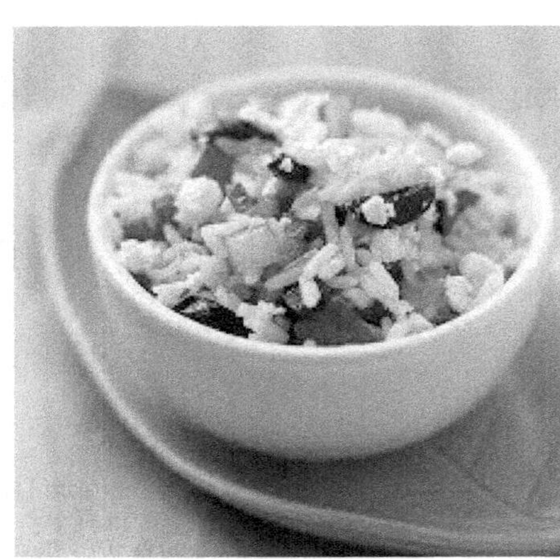

GREEK SALAD RICE

Serves: 6
Calories: 293 per serving

Ingredients

- 2 cups brown rice, cooked
- juice of 1/2 lemon
- 10 cherry tomatoes, halved
- 1/3 red onion, diced
- ½ cucumber, diced
- 2 tsp extra virgin olive oil
- 1 tsp balsamic vinegar
- 1 tsp dried oregano

Directions

1. Cook brown rice to package directions, mix in dried oregano. Set aside.

2. Prepare vegetables. Wash, dry, and cut tomatoes, and cucumbers. Cut the onion.

3. Add to a large bowl with cooled off rice, mix until combined.

4. Add olive oil, balsamic vinegar, and lemon juice over top. Just it one more toss.

5. Plate, serve, and enjoy!

Day 2

Shopping list

- Tofu
- Non-dairy milk
- Onion
- Jalapeno
- Tomatoes
- Cilantro
- Potato
- Tortilla wraps
- Chili powder
- Salt and pepper
- Lemon juice
- Lime juice
- Clove garlic
- Avocado
- Black beans
- Cumin
- Chili powder
- Garlic powder
- Portobello mushroom caps
- Red bell pepper
- Orange bell pepper
- Salt and pepper
- Virgin olive oil

BREAKFAST RECIPE

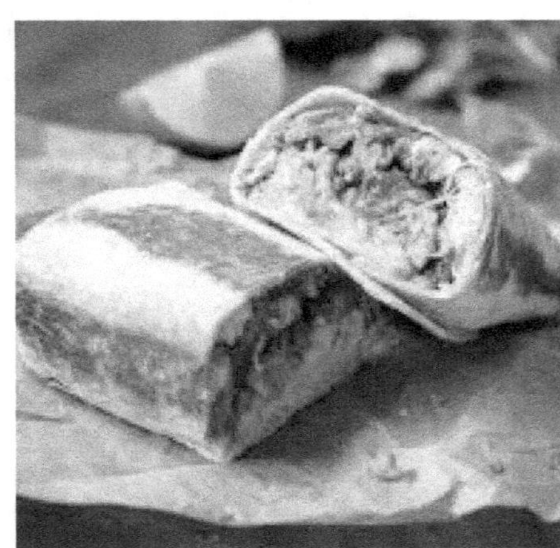

HEARTY BREAKFAST WRAP

Serves: 2
Calories: 310 per serving

Ingredients

- 1 cup extra firm tofu
- 2 tbsp plain unsweetened non-dairy milk of your choice
- ¼ onion, diced
- ¼ jalapeno, diced
- ½ tomato, diced
- ¼ cup cilantro, chopped
- 1 large potato
- 2 tortilla wraps
- 1 tsp chili powder
- 1 tsp onion powder
- pinch of salt and pepper
- 1 tsp lemon juice
- 1 tsp lime juice
- 1 clove garlic, minced

Directions

1. Prepare salsa. Wash, dry, and cut tomatoes, cilantro, and jalapeno. Cut onion and garlic. Juice lemon and lime. Combine vegetables with lemon juice, and lime juice. Mix together well and set aside.

2. Prepare potatoes. Wash, peel, and cut potatoes. The smaller you cut the potatoes the faster they will cook. Add to pan on medium heat, seasoning with a pinch of salt and pepper. Set aside.

3. Prepare tofu scramble. Drain, pat dry, and crumble extra firm tofu. Heat olive oil in the pan on medium heat. Add the crumbled tofu, chili powder, and onion powder. Add plant-based milk and cook for another minute or two until done.

4. Lay out tortillas. Spoon on the scramble, potatoes, and salsa. Wrap, serve, and enjoy!

LUNCH RECIPE

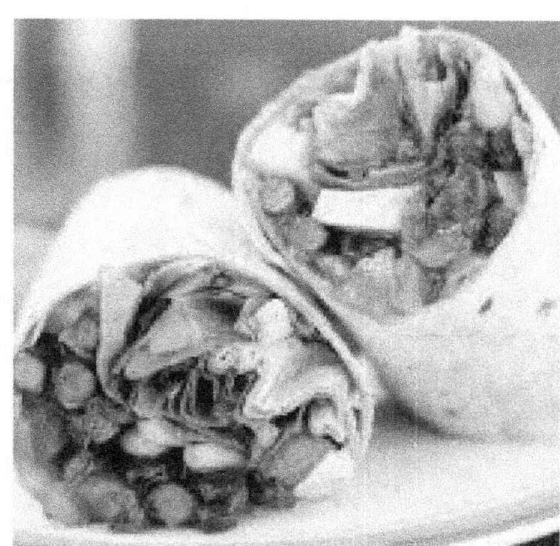

AVOCADO AND BLACK BEAN WRAP

Serves: 2
Calories: 450 per serving

Ingredients

- 1 avocado, sliced
- 2 tortilla wraps
- 1 can black beans
- 1 tomato, diced
- 1/2 tsp cumin
- ½ tsp chili powder
- ½ tsp garlic powder
- ½ tsp onion powder

Directions

1. Drain and rinse beans.
2. Warm skillet to medium heat and add beans, cumin, garlic powder, onion powder, and chili powder.
3. Stir frequently until beans are warmed through.
4. Cut avocado and tomatoes.
5. Allow beans to cool for a moment. Add to wraps. Place tomatoes and avocado on top. Wrap, serve, and enjoy!

DINNER RECIPE

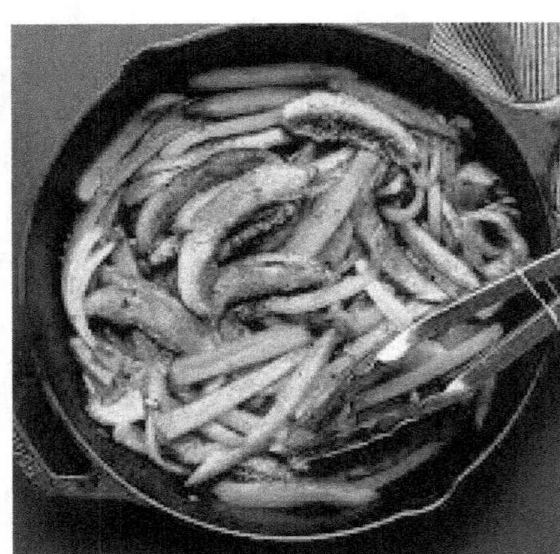

PORTOBELLO MUSHROOM FAJITAS

Serves: 2
Calories: 227 per serving

Ingredients

- 2 portobello mushroom caps, cut into thick slices (to your liking)
- 1 red bell pepper
- 1 orange bell pepper
- 1 medium onion
- Pinch of salt and pepper
- 1 tsp cumin
- 1/2 tsp garlic powder
- 1 tsp onion powder
- 1 tsp chili powder
- 2 tsp extra virgin olive oil
- Tortillas

Directions

1. Wash, dry, and cut vegetables.

2. Heat olive oil in a skillet. Add onions, mushrooms, peppers, salt, pepper, garlic powder, cumin, onion powder, and chili powder. Mix well until vegetables are all coated.

3. Cook until vegetables are warmed through and cooked to your liking.

4. Add to tortilla and top with any other toppings you like; avocado, tomatoes, salsa, guacamole, vegan cheese, or vegan sour cream.

Day 3

Shopping list

- Tofu
- Non-dairy milk
- Onion
- Jalapeno
- Tomatoes
- Cilantro
- Potato
- Tortilla wraps
- Chili powder
- Salt and pepper
- Lemon juice
- Lime juice
- Clove garlic
- Avocado
- Black beans
- Cumin
- Chili powder
- Garlic powder
- Portobello mushroom caps
- Red bell pepper
- Orange bell pepper
- Salt and pepper
- Virgin olive oil
- Spinach

BREAKFAST RECIPE

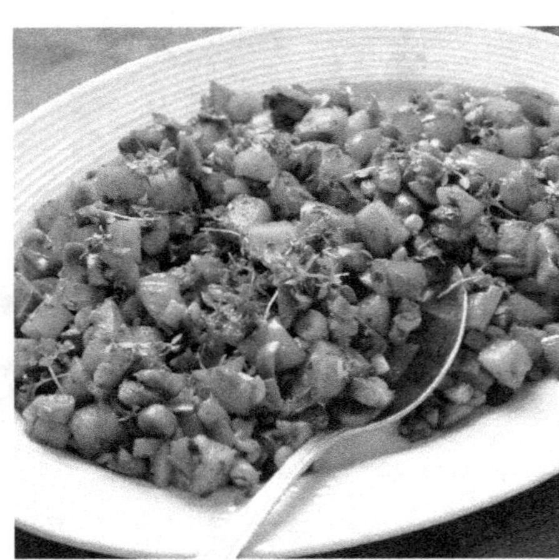

Potato Hash

Serves: 2
Calories: 308 per serving

Ingredients

- 2 large potatoes, diced
- 1 medium onion, diced
- 1 tsp extra virgin olive oil
- 1 cup mushrooms
- 1 cup spinach
- Pinch of salt and pepper
- 1 tsp garlic powder
- 1 tsp onion powder
- 1 tsp chili powder

Directions

1. Prepare vegetables; wash and cut potatoes, onion, mushrooms. Wash spinach and set all aside.

2. Heat a skillet with olive oil at medium heat. Add potatoes, and cook, stirring occasionally until tender.

3. Add onions, mushrooms, salt, pepper, garlic powder, chili powder, and onion powder. Cook until onions are tender, stirring often.

4. Add spinach, cook until wilted to your liking.

5. Let cool for a couple of minutes. Plate, serve, and enjoy!

LUNCH RECIPE

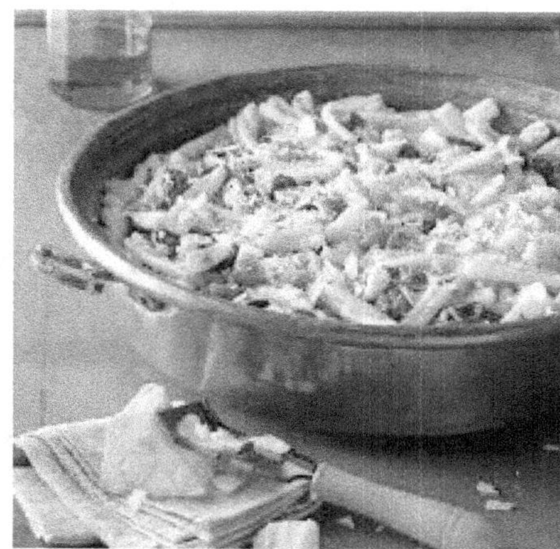

One Pot Basil and Vegetable Pasta

Serves: 8
Calories: 196 per serving

Ingredients

- 1 lbs package of pasta of your choice
- 1 bunch basil, stems removed
- Pinch of salt and pepper
- 3 cloves of garlic, minced
- 1 red bell pepper, sliced
- 8 asparagus, cut into pieces
- 1 cup mushrooms, sliced
- 1 onion, diced
- 1 tbsp olive oil (roughly, may need more or less as per your liking)

Directions

1. Combine onion, garlic, basil, pepper, and asparagus and add water. Bring to a boil.

2. Cover pot and allow to boil for 10 minutes or until pasta is done.

3. Drain water. Add mushrooms to pasta and mix with the heat on medium.

4. Add olive oil, salt, and pepper. Toss to evenly coat all of the pasta and allow the mushrooms to warm through.

5. Plate, serve, and enjoy!

DINNER RECIPE

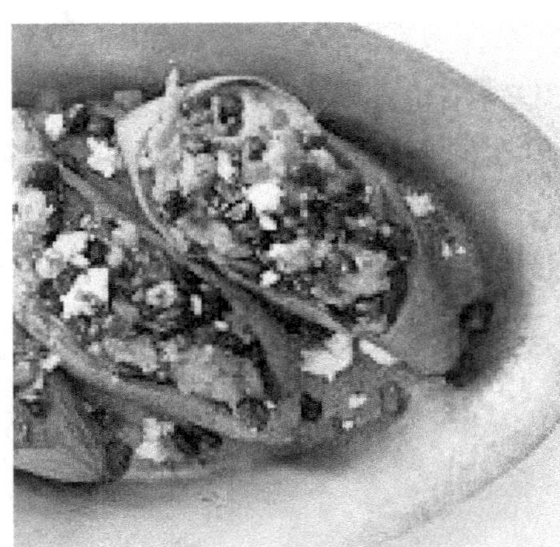

LOADED SWEET POTATOES

Serves: 2
Calories: 456 per serving

Ingredients

- 2 medium sweet potatoes
- 1 can black beans
- 1 tsp cumin
- 1 tsp garlic powder
- 1 tsp chili powder
- 1 tsp onion powder
- 1 medium tomato, diced
- 1/2 medium onion, diced
- 1 cup of corn

Directions

1. Preheat oven to 400 °F.

2. Prepare sweet potato. Wash, dry, pierce with fork and place on a baking sheet. Cooking for 40 minutes or until done.

3. In a skillet heat a small amount of olive oil over medium heat. Add black beans, corn, onion cumin, garlic powder, chili powder, and onion powder. Stirring frequently until thoroughly warmed through and onions go soft.

4. Prepare tomato; wash, dry, cut.

5. When sweet potatoes are finished. Cut them lengthwise and serve on a plate. Pour the bean mixture over the sweet potatoes. Plate, serve, and enjoy!

Day 4

Shopping list

- Tofu
- Non-dairy milk
- Onion
- Jalapeno
- Tomatoes
- Cilantro
- Potato
- Tortilla wraps
- Chili powder
- Salt and pepper
- Lemon juice
- Lime juice
- Clove garlic
- Avocado
- Black beans
- Cumin
- Chili powder
- Garlic powder
- Portobello mushroom caps
- Red bell pepper
- Orange bell pepper
- Salt and pepper
- Virgin olive oil
- Spinach
- Potatoes
- Spinach
- Parsley
- Carrots
- Vegetable broth

BREAKFAST RECIPE

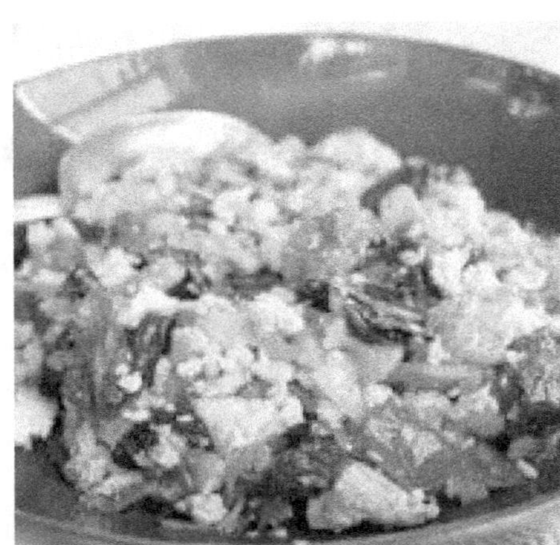

TOFU SCRAMBLE WITH VEGETABLES

Serves: 2
Calories: 300 per serving

Ingredients

- ¾ cup extra firm tofu
- pinch of salt and pepper
- garlic powder
- onion powder
- 1 tsp extra virgin olive oil

- ½ bell pepper (color of your choice), diced
- ¼ onion, diced
- 2 tbsp plain unsweetened non-dairy milk of your choice

Directions

1. Prepare vegetables. Wash and cut bell pepper. Cut onion, set all aside.

2. Prepare tofu; drain, pat dry, and crumble. Stir frequently for a few minutes

3. Heat olive oil in the pan on medium heat. Add the crumbled tofu, salt, pepper, garlic powder, onion powder. Add plant-based milk and cook for another minute or two until done.

4. Add onions and peppers to the scramble. Cook stirring frequently until the vegetables are softer, to your liking. Be careful to not overcook the tofu scramble. Alternatively, you can make them in a separate pan then combine and mix.

5. Serve with some toast or on a wrap for a full breakfast. Enjoy!

LUNCH RECIPE

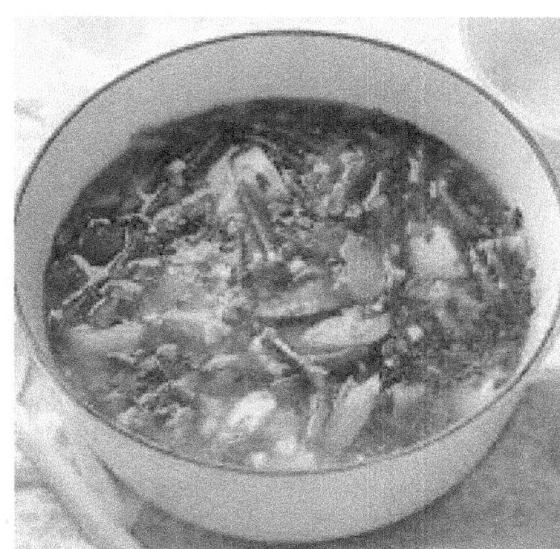

Vegetable Soup

Serves: 8
Calories: 139 per serving

Ingredients

- 2 tbsp extra virgin olive
- 4 stalks of celery, chopped
- 4 cloves of garlic, minced
- 1 onion, diced
- 2 tbsp tomato puree
- 2 tsp cumin
- 2 tsp onion powder
- 1 tsp chili powder

- 1 can stewed tomatoes
- 2 potatoes, diced
- 3 cups spinach
- 1 cup parsley, chopped
- 3 carrots, diced
- Pinch of salt and pepper
- 8 cups vegetable broth

Directions

1. Heat olive oil. Add onion, garlic, celery, and carrots. Cook until onions are tender. Stirring often.

2. Add tomato puree, salt, pepper, cumin, onion powder, and chili powder. Let cook for a couple of minutes.

3. Add potatoes, stewed tomatoes, and vegetable broth.

4. Boil for 10 minutes. Then bring down to a simmer for at 30 minutes or until potatoes are cooked through. The smaller the potatoes are cut, the faster they will cook.

5. Add spinach and parsley, stir well and frequently until spinach is wilted to your liking.

6. Let cool slightly, serve, and enjoy!

DINNER RECIPE

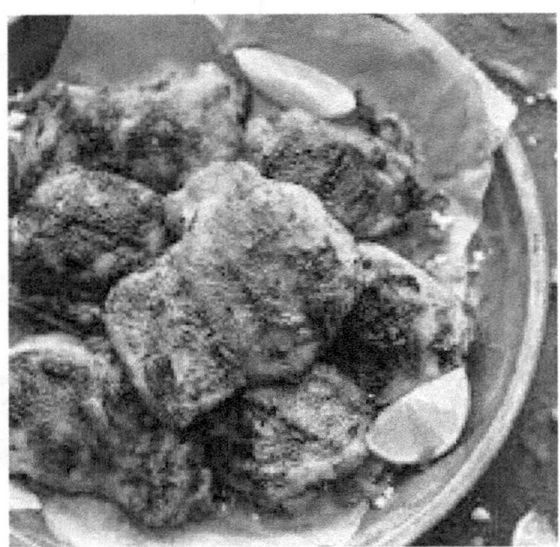

GRILLED CAJUN PINEAPPLE AND LEMON RICE

Serves: 4
Calories: 276 per serving

Ingredients

- 1 large pineapple, core and skin removed and cut into steaks
- Cajun seasoning (prepackaged or a mix of your own - chili powder, onion powder, garlic powder, a pinch of salt and pepper)
- 4 cups of brown rice, cooked
- juice of one lemon
- 3/4 cup cilantro, chopped

Directions

1. Cook rice to directions on the package but add the lemon juice to the water while cooking.

2. Chop cilantro, set aside.

3. When rice is finished, fluff with a fork and mix in cilantro.

4. Prepare pineapple, wash and remove the skin. Remove the core and cut into thick pieces. 8 pieces will be 1 serving for 4 people.

5. Mix in the cajun seasoning with olive oil and brush onto pineapple pieces.

6. Grill on medium heat for roughly 8 minutes and flip. Pineapple should still be juicy and tender but begin to brown around edges. Cook for another couple of minutes.

7. Plate the rice and pineapple, serve, and enjoy!

Day 5

Shopping list

- Tofu
- Non-dairy milk
- Onion
- Jalapeno
- Tomatoes
- Cilantro
- Potato
- Tortilla wraps
- Chili powder
- Salt and pepper
- Lemon juice
- Lime juice
- Clove garlic
- Avocado
- Black beans
- Cumin
- Chili powder
- Garlic powder
- Portobello mushroom caps
- Red bell pepper
- Orange bell pepper
- Salt and pepper
- Virgin olive oil
- Spinach
- Potatoes
- Spinach
- Parsley
- Carrots
- Vegetable broth

BREAKFAST RECIPE

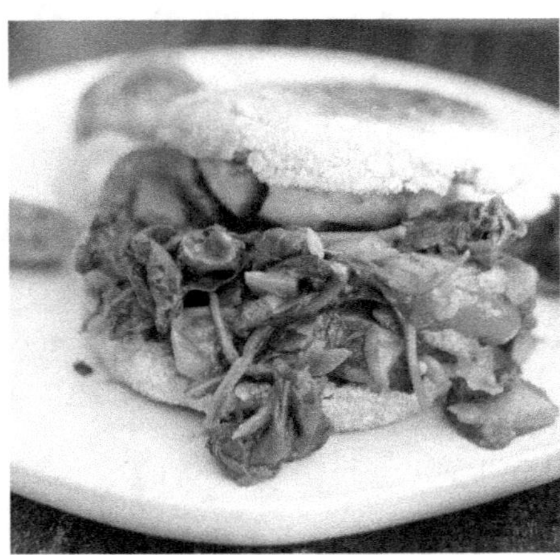

Mushroom English Muffin

Serves: 1
Calories: 194 per serving

Ingredients

- 3 cremini mushrooms, sliced
- 1 slice of red onion
- 1/4 cup spinach
- 1 slice of tomato
- Pinch of salt and pepper
- Pinch of red pepper flakes
- English muffin
- 1 tsp extra virgin olive oil

Directions

1. Clean dirt off of mushrooms with a damp paper towel and slice them.

2. Wash, dry, and cut tomato. Slice red onion. Wash spinach. Set all aside.

3. Warm olive oil over medium heat in a skillet. Place mushroom slices in skillet and season with salt, pepper, and red pepper flakes. Stirring frequently to cook.

4. Toast English muffin.

5. Place mushrooms, spinach, tomato, and onion on English muffin.

6. Plate, serve and enjoy!

LUNCH RECIPE

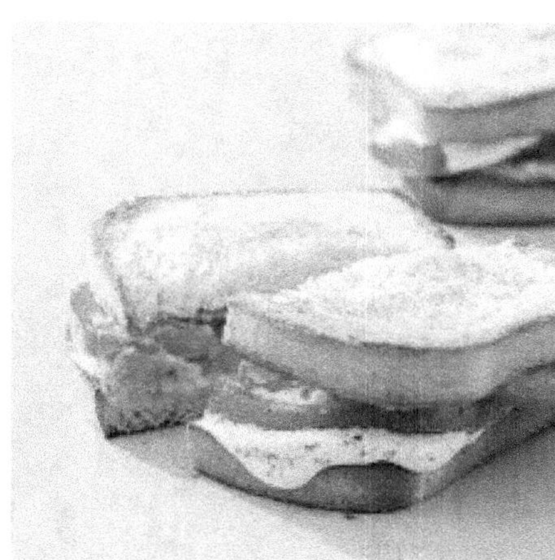

TOMATO SANDWICH

Serves: 1
Calories: 170 per serving

Ingredients

- ½ a large tomato
- pinch of salt and pepper
- 1 tbsp hummus
- 2 slices of whole grain bread

Directions

1. Wash, dry, and cut tomatoes. Slice to your preferred thickness.
2. Toast bread to your liking.
3. Spoon hummus over one side, add tomato on top, sprinkle salt and pepper to your liking.
4. Cut in half, serve and enjoy!

DINNER RECIPE

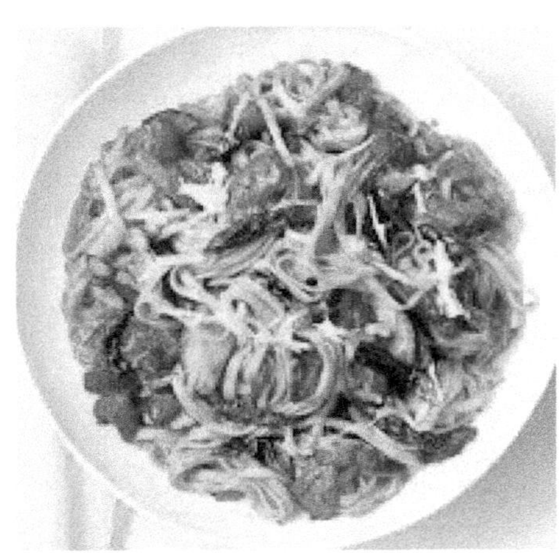

ROASTED VEGETABLE PASTA

Serves: 3
Calories: 353 per serving

Ingredients

- Package of pasta, roughly 6 oz
- 1 large zucchini
- 1 medium red onion
- 1 cup of corn
- 1 bell pepper
- Extra virgin olive oil
- ½ cup of basil, chopped

Directions

1. Preheat oven to 375 °F.

2. Prepare vegetables; wash, dry, cut, and place on the baking sheet. Bake until done, roughly 45 minutes.

3. While vegetables are roasting to cook the pasta. Cook for roughly 10 minutes or until pasta is done.

4. Drain the pasta and put back into the large pot.

5. When vegetables are cooked, take them out of the oven and add them to the large pot.

6. Add a drizzle of olive oil, salt, pepper, and basil. Toss until well combined.

7. Plate, serve, and enjoy!

Day 6

Shopping list

- Tofu
- Non-dairy milk
- Onion
- Jalapeno
- Tomatoes
- Cilantro
- Potato
- Tortilla wraps
- Chili powder
- Salt and pepper
- Lemon juice
- Lime juice
- Clove garlic
- Avocado
- Black beans
- Cumin
- Chili powder
- Garlic powder
- Portobello mushroom caps
- Red bell pepper
- Orange bell pepper
- Salt and pepper
- Virgin olive oil
- Spinach
- Potatoes
- Spinach
- Parsley
- Carrots
- Vegetable broth

BREAKFAST RECIPE

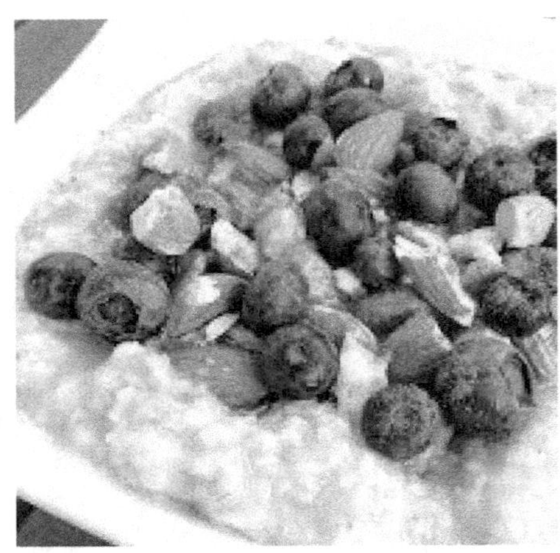

BERRY ALMOND STEEL CUT OATS

Serves: 1
Calories: 358 per serving

Ingredients

- 1 cup steel cut oats, cooked
- Splash of unsweetened vanilla almond milk
- 1/2 tsp cinnamon
- 1/4 cup strawberries, diced
- 1/4 cup blueberries
- 1/4 cup raspberries
- a drizzle of maple syrup

Directions

1. Cook steel cut oats to package directions. You're going to want about 1 cup of cooked oats for a serving.

2. Prepare fruit. Wash, dry, cut berries, set aside.

3. Put oats in a serving bowl, add a splash of almond milk, and a drizzle of maple syrup over top, both to your liking.

4. Sprinkle cinnamon on top with the berries. Serve and enjoy!

LUNCH RECIPE

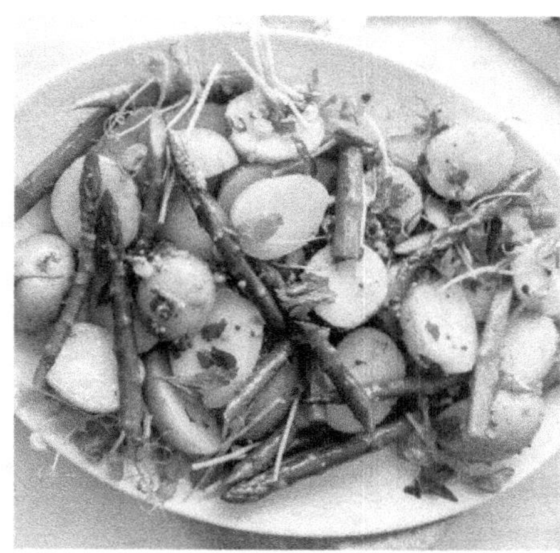

Warm Potato Salad

Serves: 4
Calories: 191 per serving

Ingredients

- 4 potatoes, diced
- 1 cup green onions, sliced
- 1 tbsp extra virgin olive oil
- Pinch of salt and pepper
- 8 asparagus, cut into pieces
- balsamic vinegar

Directions

1. Wash, dry, and cut potatoes.
2. Boil in salted water.
3. Prepare asparagus and green onion, wash, dry, cut.
4. Heat olive oil. Add asparagus and stir frequently until cooked to your liking.
5. When done add to the bowl of potatoes and add the green onion.
6. Add a drizzle of extra virgin olive oil and balsamic vinegar, gently toss until combined.
7. Plate and serve warm. Enjoy!

DINNER RECIPE

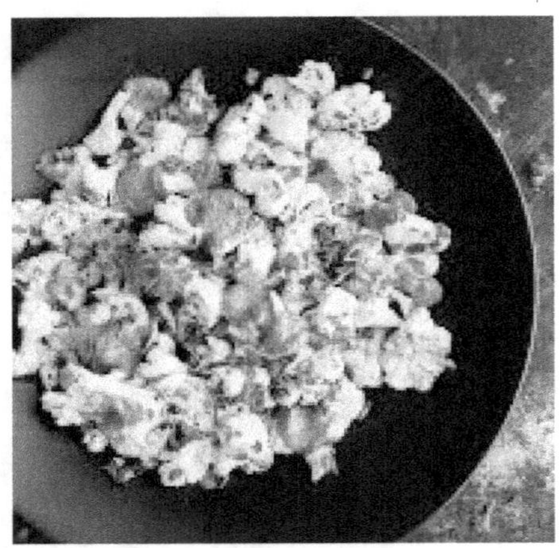

Roasted Cauliflower with Chimichurri Sauce

Serves: 2
Calories: 299 per serving

Ingredients

- 1 large head of cauliflower
- 3 tbsp extra virgin olive oil
- 1/3 cup cilantro, chopped
- 1/3 cup parsley, chopped

- 2 tbsp red wine vinegar
- 1 jalapeno, seeds removed, finely chopped
- 2 cloves of garlic, minced
- pinch of salt and pepper

Directions

1. Preheat oven to 425°F.

2. Wash, dry, and cut cauliflower. Put in a bowl. Toss with roughly 2 tbsp oil, salt, and pepper. You want just enough oil to coat the cauliflower lightly and evenly. Add little bits at a time to not over add.

3. Put cauliflower on a baking sheet. Bake for 20 minutes, flip, and bake another 5 minutes or until done.

4. Make the sauce by mixing the cilantro, 2 tbsp oil, parsley, garlic, vinegar, jalapeno, and a small pinch of salt.

5. When cauliflower is done, plate and pour the sauce over them. Serve and enjoy!

Day 7

Shopping list

- Tofu
- Non-dairy milk
- Onion
- Jalapeno
- Tomatoes
- Cilantro
- Potato
- Tortilla wraps
- Chili powder
- Salt and pepper
- Lemon juice
- Lime juice
- Clove garlic
- Avocado
- Black beans
- Cumin
- Chili powder
- Garlic powder
- Portobello mushroom caps
- Red bell pepper
- Orange bell pepper
- Salt and pepper
- Virgin olive oil
- Spinach
- Potatoes
- Spinach
- Parsley
- Carrots
- Vegetable broth

BREAKFAST RECIPE

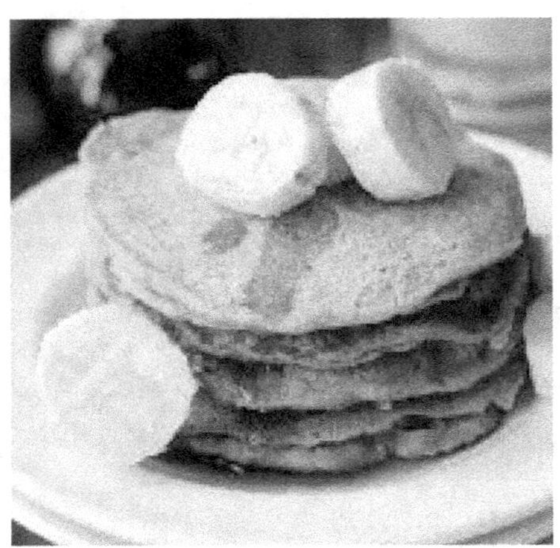

Banana Pumpkin Pie Pancakes

Serves: 4
Calories: 345 per serving

Ingredients

- 3 cups oat flour
- 1 1/2 tsp pumpkin pie spice
- 2 cups unsweetened vanilla almond milk
- 2 overripe bananas

Directions

1. Mash bananas in a large bowl
2. Add flour, pumpkin pie spice, and almond milk. Use a hand mixer and mix until batter forms.
3. Heat non-stick skillet on medium.
4. Pour batter in equal parts into the skillet. You can use a measuring cup to ensure size consistency. 1/3 cup measuring cup works best.
5. Once bubbles begin to form over the top of the pancakes and the edges are set, flip the cake and cook until golden.
6. Plate and top with some more bananas, a drizzle of maple syrup, or whatever you prefer. Serve and enjoy!

LUNCH RECIPE

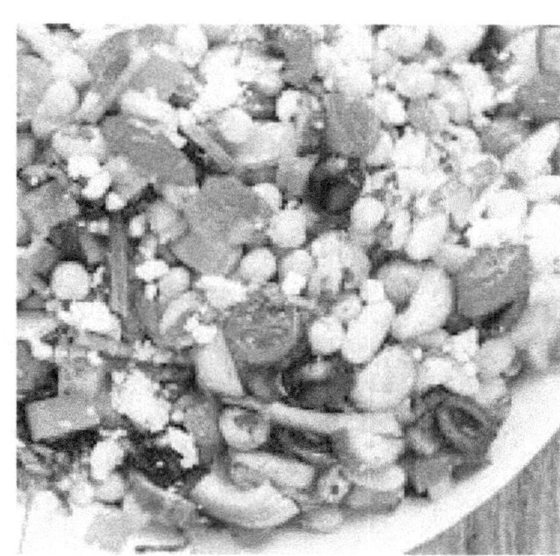

Bean Salad

Serves: 4
Calories: 200 per serving

Ingredients

- 1 can mixed beans
- ½ large red onion, diced
- 4 stalks of celery
- 1 large tomato, diced and seeds removed
- ½ large English cucumber, diced
- 2 large carrots, shredded

Directions

1. Drain and rinse beans, add them to a large bowl.
2. Cut onion add to bowl.
3. Wash, dry, and cut the celery, tomatoes, and cucumber. Wash, dry, and shred the carrots. Add all to bowl.
4. Add dressing, toss gently until mixed well.
5. Serve and enjoy!

DINNER RECIPE

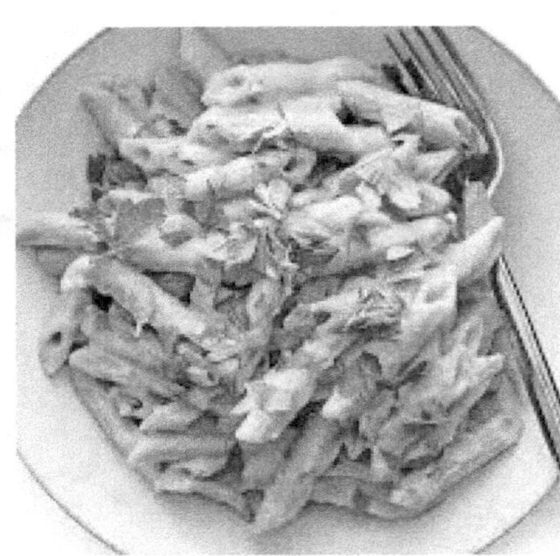

CHICKPEA PASTA

Serves: 3
Calories: 496 per serving

Ingredients

- ½ onion, diced
- 1 package chickpea pasta
- 3 cloves garlic, minced
- 1 zucchini, diced
- 2 carrots, diced
- 1 eggplant, diced
- 1 large can chopped tomatoes (about 400 g)
- ½ cup basil, chopped
- 1 can tomato or pasta sauce

Directions

1. Cook chickpea pasta to directions. Drain.
2. Heat olive oil in a skillet over medium heat. Add onions, garlic, zucchini, eggplant, and carrots. Allow them to cook while frequently stirring.
3. Add tomatoes, tomato sauce, basil, and pasta.
4. Stir and heat through.
5. Plate, serve, and enjoy!

Day 8

Shopping list

- Tofu
- Non-dairy milk
- Onion
- Jalapeno
- Tomatoes
- Cilantro
- Potato
- Tortilla wraps
- Chili powder
- Salt and pepper
- Lemon juice
- Lime juice
- Clove garlic
- Avocado
- Black beans
- Cumin
- Chili powder
- Garlic powder
- Portobello mushroom caps
- Red bell pepper
- Orange bell pepper
- Salt and pepper
- Virgin olive oil
- Spinach
- Potatoes
- Spinach
- Parsley
- Carrots
- Vegetable broth

BREAKFAST RECIPE

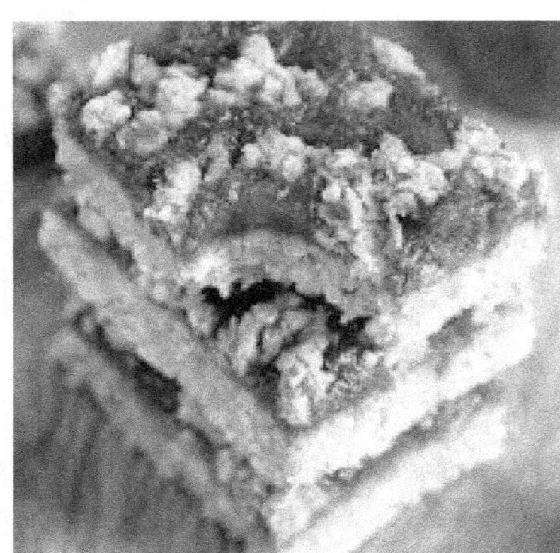

BANANA STRAWBERRY BARS

Serves: 12
Calories: 165 per serving

Ingredients

- 2 ripe bananas
- 1 ½ cups dates, pitted
- 3 cups rolled oats
- ½ tsp cinnamon
- ½ tsp nutmeg
- 1/4 tsp cardamom
- 1 ½ tbsp baking powder
- 1 1/2 tsp vanilla extract
- 1 cup strawberries, diced

Directions

1. Preheat the oven to 375 °F.
2. Line a 9x9 inch baking pan with parchment paper, placing paper over the sides as well.
3. In a bowl mix half of the oats, vanilla, nutmeg, cinnamon, cardamom, and baking powder together. Set aside.
4. In a blender blend together the rest of the oats, bananas, a splash of vanilla, and the apple juice (without the dates) until smooth
5. Add dates and blend for a moment until they are to your liking.
6. Add the strawberries into the mixture and pour it onto the baking pan.
7. Bake for roughly 30-40 minutes until cooked through.
8. Allow to cool and cut into 12. Serve and enjoy!

LUNCH RECIPE

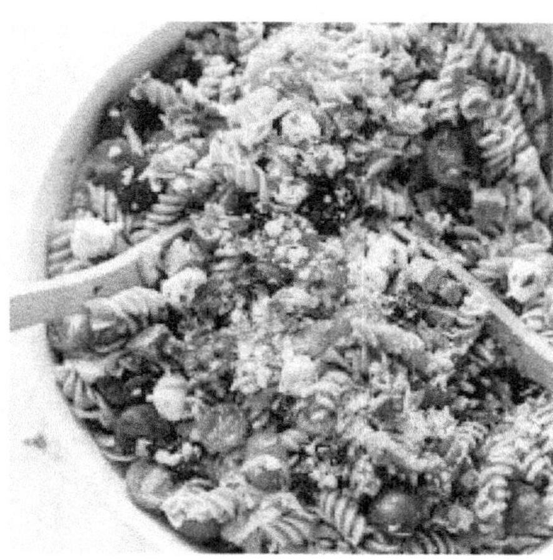

Pasta Salad

Serves: 6
Calories: 400 per serving

Ingredients

- 1 package of pasta
- 1 head of broccoli, chopped
- ½ red onion, diced
- 1 bell pepper, diced
- ½ can of black olives, halved
- 4 tbsp zesty Italian dressing

Directions

1. Cook pasta, drain. Add a splash of dressing and mix to stop the pasta from sticking together. Set aside in a large bowl in the refrigerator. Let cool completely.

2. Wash, dry, and cut broccoli and bell pepper. Add to pasta.

3. Cut onion and olives and add to pasta.

4. Pour in dressing and mix a little bit at a time, to your liking.

5. Serve and enjoy!

DINNER RECIPE

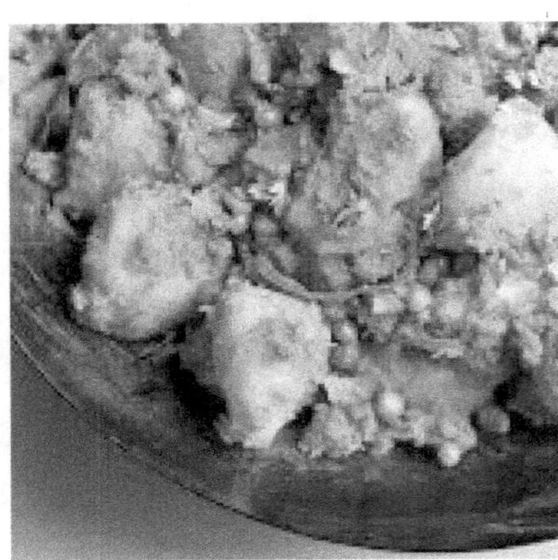

Potato and Pea Curry

Serves: 4
Calories: 320 Per Serving

Ingredients

- 3 large potatoes
- 3 cloves garlic, minced
- 1 tbsp cumin
- 1 tbsp chili powder
- 1 cup coriander, chopped
- pinch of salt and pepper
- 3 tbsp vegetable oil
- 2 cups of water
- 1/2 onion, diced
- 1 cup of peas

Directions

1. Prepare potatoes; wash, peel, dry, and cut into small cubes.
2. Cook, stirring frequently for a minute.
3. Add potatoes, cook for a few minutes.
4. Add in cumin, chili, salt, and pepper. Stirring well. Add water, potatoes should be almost covered by the water. Add peas, frozen works best.
5. Potatoes should be cooked all the way through, check to see if they are cooked. If not after 20 minutes you may add another cup of water and cook again.
6. When the curry is done, and the right consistency and the potatoes are fully cooked add in the coriander and cook for a couple of minutes.
7. Plate, serve with rice or bread, and enjoy!

Day 9

Shopping list

- Tofu
- Non-dairy milk
- Onion
- Jalapeno
- Tomatoes
- Cilantro
- Potato
- Tortilla wraps
- Chili powder
- Salt and pepper
- Lemon juice
- Lime juice
- Clove garlic
- Avocado
- Black beans
- Cumin
- Chili powder
- Garlic powder
- Portobello mushroom caps
- Red bell pepper
- Orange bell pepper
- Salt and pepper
- Virgin olive oil
- Spinach
- Potatoes
- Spinach
- Parsley
- Carrots
- Vegetable broth

BREAKFAST RECIPE

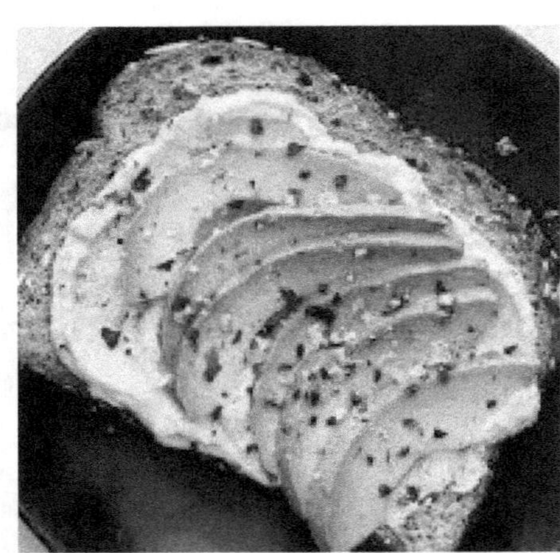

HUMMUS AND AVOCADO TOAST

Serves: 2
Calories: 247 per serving

Ingredients

- 2 pieces of whole grain bread
- 1 tbsp hummus
- ½ half an avocado, cut into slices
- ½ a tomato, cut into slices
- pinch of salt and pepper

Directions

1. Prepare vegetables; wash, dry, and cut tomato and avocado.

2. Toast bread to your liking.

3. Spread hummus over each slice of bread, place slices of tomato over the hummus and add a pinch of salt and pepper.

4. Top each piece of bread with avocado. Serve and enjoy!

LUNCH RECIPE

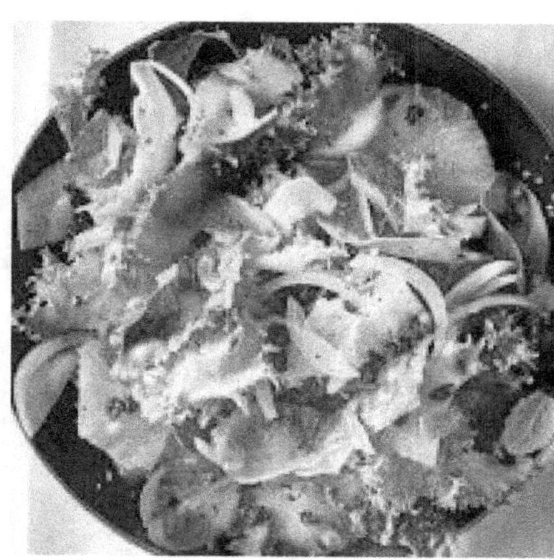

Citrus Salad

Serves: 4
Calories: 301 per serving

Ingredients

- 4 cups spinach
- ½ small red onion, diced
- 1 medium mandarin orange
- ½ a grapefruit
- 1 tbsp lemon juice
- 1 can chickpeas

Directions

1. Wash spinach, place in a large bowl.
2. Cut onion, peel orange and grapefruit, cut segments in half and add to spinach bowl.
3. Drain and rinse chickpeas.
4. Add lemon juice and toss gently.
5. Plate, serve, and enjoy!

DINNER RECIPE

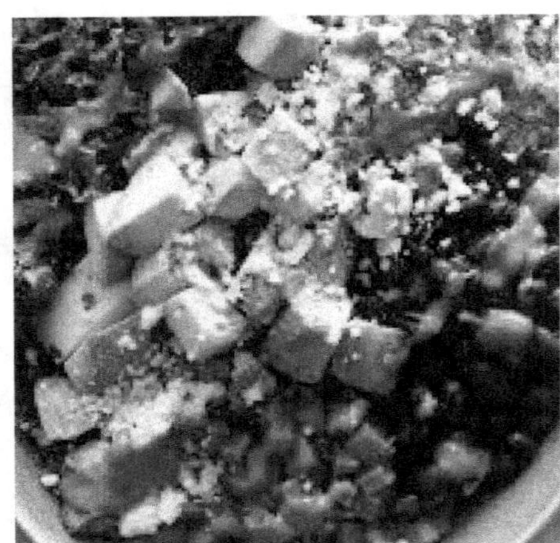

SWEET POTATO SOUTHWEST BOWL

Serves: 3
Calories: 317 per serving

Ingredients

- 1 sweet potato, cut into cubes
- 1 cup brown rice, cooked
- 1/3 cup cilantro, chopped
- 1 cup corn, cooked but not warm
- 1/3 medium onion, chopped
- 1/3 jalapeno, chopped, seeds removed
- 1/3 large tomato, chopped, seeds removed
- 1 tsp cumin
- 1/2 tsp garlic powder
- 1 tsp onion powder
- 1 tsp chili powder
- extra virgin olive oil

Directions

1. Preheat oven to 375 °F.
2. Wash, peel, cut sweet potatoes. Place on a baking sheet in single layer and bake 30 minutes or until done.
3. While sweet potatoes are cooking, cook rice to directions on the package.
4. Heat a little olive oil, roughly a tsp just to coat the bottom, on medium heat in a skillet. Drain and rinse.
5. Add cumin, garlic powder, onion powder, chili powder, salt, and pepper to taste. Stirring frequently until beans are coated and warmed all the way through.
6. Wash, dry, and cut tomatoes, cilantro, and jalapenos. Mix in a small bowl with onion and corn.
7. Place rice in a bowl, add sweet potato on top, beans next to them, and corn salsa beside them both.
8. Serve and enjoy!

Day 10

Shopping list

- Tofu
- Non-dairy milk
- Onion
- Jalapeno
- Tomatoes
- Cilantro
- Potato
- Tortilla wraps
- Chili powder
- Salt and pepper
- Lemon juice
- Lime juice
- Clove garlic
- Avocado
- Black beans
- Cumin
- Chili powder
- Garlic powder
- Portobello mushroom caps
- Red bell pepper
- Orange bell pepper
- Salt and pepper
- Virgin olive oil
- Spinach
- Potatoes
- Spinach
- Parsley
- Carrots
- Vegetable broth

BREAKFAST RECIPE

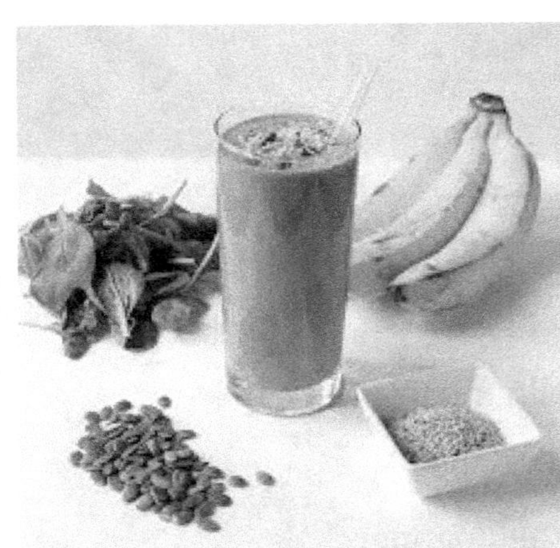

POWER BREAKFAST SMOOTHIE

Serves: 1
Calories: 377 per serving

Ingredients

- 1 1/2 cups spinach
- 1 banana
- 1 small apple
- 1 cup of orange juice
- 1 tsp ginger root, minced
- 1 tbsp chia seeds

Directions

1. Prepare ingredients; wash and cut apple, peel a banana, wash spinach, and mince ginger. Place them all into your blender.

2. Add orange juice and chia seeds

3. Blend until smooth. Serve and enjoy!

LUNCH RECIPE

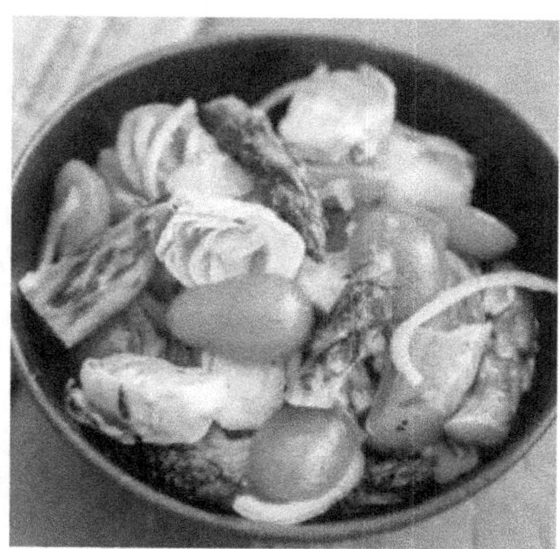

Asparagus and Artichoke Salad

Serves: 8
Prep time: 1 hour and 5 minutes

Ingredients

- 20 tender, fresh green asparagus stalks (woody stem removed, rinsed)
- 8 fresh, medium artichokes
- 4 tablespoons extra virgin olive oil
- 2 cloves garlic, peeled and chopped
- 1 ounce chopped pistachio nuts
- 1 large egg white
- 4 teaspoons chopped green onions + 1 green onion for garnish, chopped
- Juice of 1 lemon
- Salt and white pepper to taste

Directions

1. Fill a large pot ¾ of the way with water; add half the lemon juice and a generous sprinkle of salt.

2. Trim the artichokes by removing the leaves until you get to the light-yellow leaves. Set the hearts aside.

3. Place the artichoke leaves in boiling water. Cook 45 minutes. Once boiled, rinse under cold water.

4. Place the artichoke leaves in a food processor. Add the remaining lemon juice, half a glass of water (4 ounces), pinch of salt and pepper, pistachios, green onions, garlic, and egg white. Blend for 1 minute. Add the olive oil slowly. Continue to blend until smooth.

5. Cut up the artichoke hearts and arrange on plate. Place the asparagus over top. Drizzle the sauce over the artichokes and asparagus. Garnish with fresh green onions. Serve.

Nutritional Value (Amount per Serving)

Protein   5.9 g
Carbs: 11 g
Fat: 7 g

DINNER RECIPE

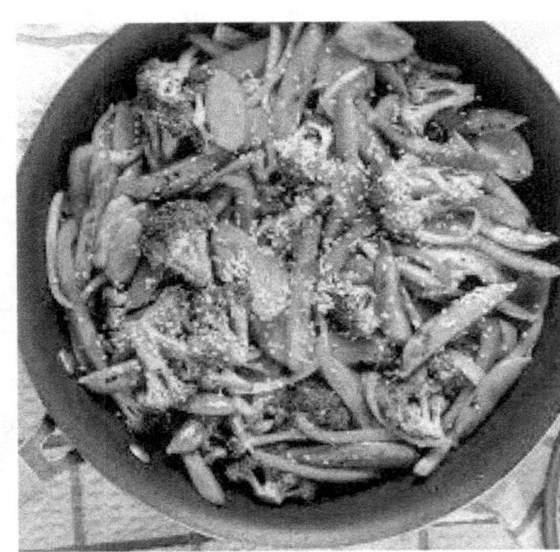

VEGETABLE STIR FRY

Serves: 4
Calories: 428 per serving

Another great classic that even the kids will be asking for seconds. Stir fry is cheap, easy, fast, and easily changed up how you like. Perfect for lunch or dinner.

Ingredients

- 2 cups brown rice, cooked
- 1 cup mushrooms, sliced
- 1 cup snap peas
- 1 medium onion, chopped
- 1 bell pepper
- 1 tbsp soy sauce
- 2 tsp cooking oil of your choice
- 1/3 cup water chestnuts, sliced
- 1 tbsp grated ginger

Directions

1. Cook brown rice, set aside
2. Prepare vegetables; wash, dry, cut. Grate ginger and set aside.

Day 11

Shopping list

- Tofu
- Non-dairy milk
- Onion
- Jalapeno
- Tomatoes
- Cilantro
- Potato
- Tortilla wraps
- Chili powder
- Salt and pepper
- Lemon juice
- Lime juice
- Clove garlic
- Avocado
- Black beans
- Cumin
- Chili powder
- Garlic powder
- Portobello mushroom caps
- Red bell pepper
- Orange bell pepper
- Salt and pepper
- Virgin olive oil
- Spinach
- Potatoes
- Spinach
- Parsley
- Carrots
- Vegetable broth

BREAKFAST RECIPE

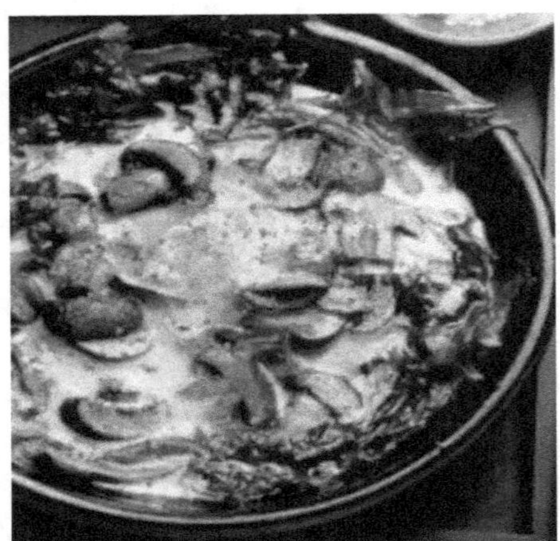

Baked Eggs with Spinach and Mushrooms

Serves: 3
Prep time: 20 minutes

Ingredients

- 4 large eggs
- 3 cups chopped spinach
- 3 cups sliced mushrooms
- 1 green bell pepper, coarsely chopped
- 2 tablespoons extra virgin olive oil
- Salt and pepper to taste

Directions

1. Preheat oven to 400□F. Grease an 8x8 baking dish with olive oil.
2. Place the bell peppers, spinach, and mushrooms in the baking dish.
3. Carefully crack the eggs over the vegetables. Season with salt and pepper.
4. Bake until the whites are set, approximately 10 minutes.
5. Transfer to plates. Serve.

Nutritional Value (Amount per Serving)

Protein: 12.7 g
Carbs: 7.6 g
Fat: 9.9 g

LUNCH RECIPE

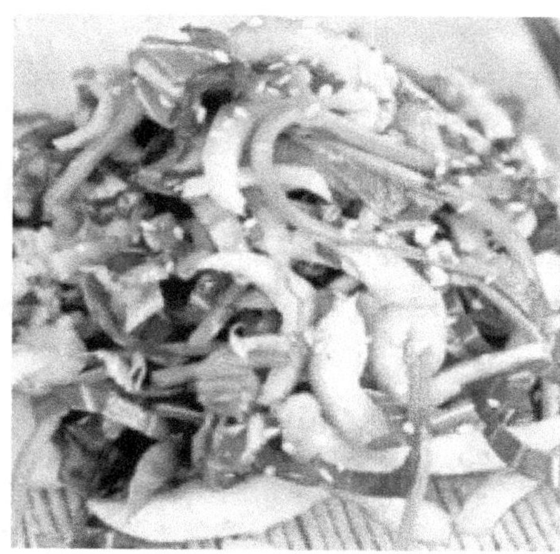

Pressure-Cooker Bok Choy Warm Salad

Serves: 3
Prep time: 10 minutes

Ingredients

- 1 bunch trimmed bok choy
- 2 cups water
- 2 tablespoons olive oil
- 2 tablespoons fresh-squeezed lime juice
- Salt and pepper to taste

Directions

1. Place the bok choy in the pressure cooker. Add enough water to cover.
2. Close lid. Set pressure to High. Cook 7 minutes.
3. Once cooked, allow the pressure to drop naturally, approximately 20 minutes.
4. Transfer to a serving platter. Drizzle lime juice and oil over. Sprinkle with salt and pepper. Serve.

Nutritional Value (Amount per Serving)

Protein: 8.5 g
Carbs: 9.9 g
Fat: 10.1 g

DINNER RECIPE

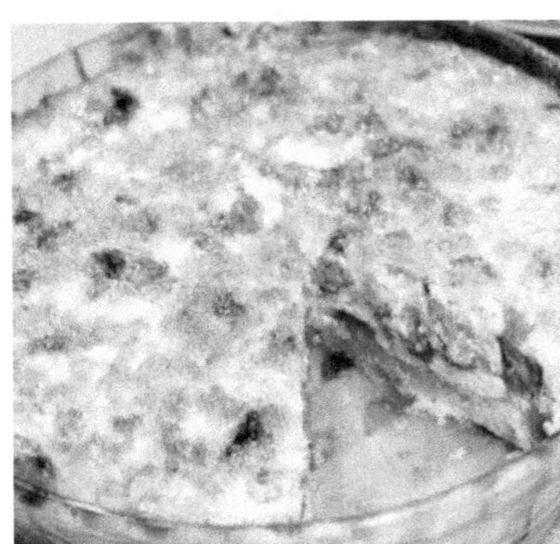

Crustless Feta Mushroom Quiche

Serves: 6
Prep time: 45 minutes

Ingredients

- 8 ounces' button mushrooms, thinly sliced
- 1 clove garlic, minced
- 10 ounces thawed frozen spinach
- 4 large eggs
- 1 cup milk
- 2 ounces' feta cheese
- ¼ cup grated Parmesan
- ½ cup shredded mozzarella
- Salt & pepper to taste

Directions

1. Preheat oven to 400°F. Squeeze excess water out of the thawed spinach.

2. Heat a tablespoon or so of cooking oil in a large non-stick frying pan over medium heat.

3. Add the garlic and mushrooms. Sauté until tender, approximately 7 minutes.

4. Grease a large pie dish with non-stick spray. Arrange the spinach along the bottom of the pie dish. Pour the mushrooms and garlic over the spinach. Crumble feta cheese over top.

5. In a large bowl, whisk together the milk, eggs, and Parmesan cheese. Lightly season with pepper. Pour the egg mixture on top of the ingredients in the pie dish.

6. Sprinkle mozzarella over the top.

Nutritional Value (Amount per Serving)

Protein: 17 g
Carbs: 4 g
Fat: 18 g

Day 12

Shopping list

- Tofu
- Non-dairy milk
- Onion
- Jalapeno
- Tomatoes
- Cilantro
- Potato
- Tortilla wraps
- Chili powder
- Salt and pepper
- Lemon juice
- Lime juice
- Clove garlic
- Avocado
- Black beans
- Cumin
- Chili powder
- Garlic powder
- Portobello mushroom caps
- Red bell pepper
- Orange bell pepper
- Salt and pepper
- Virgin olive oil
- Spinach
- Potatoes
- Spinach
- Parsley
- Carrots
- Vegetable broth

BREAKFAST RECIPE

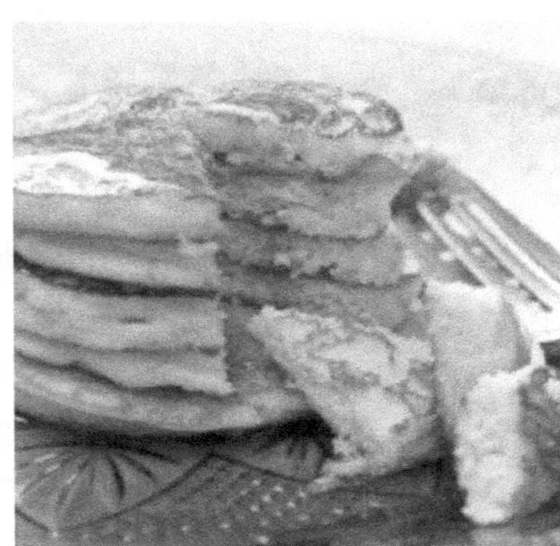

FLAXSEED COTTAGE PANCAKES

Serves: 6
Prep time: 15 minutes

Ingredients

- ½ cup ground flax seed meal
- 3 tablespoons cottage cheese
- 2 large eggs
- 2 tablespoons butter
- ½ cup heavy cream
- ¼ teaspoon gluten-free baking powder
- Coconut oil or olive oil for frying

Directions

1. Combine all the ingredients. Whisk together thoroughly.
2. Heat the oil.
3. Spoon ¾ cup of batter into the frying pan. Cook for 2 minutes per side.
4. Transfer onto plate. Serve with fresh berries or (keto-friendly) syrup.

Nutritional Value (Amount per Serving)

Protein: 6.1 g
Carbs: 4.5 g
Fat: 13 g

LUNCH RECIPE

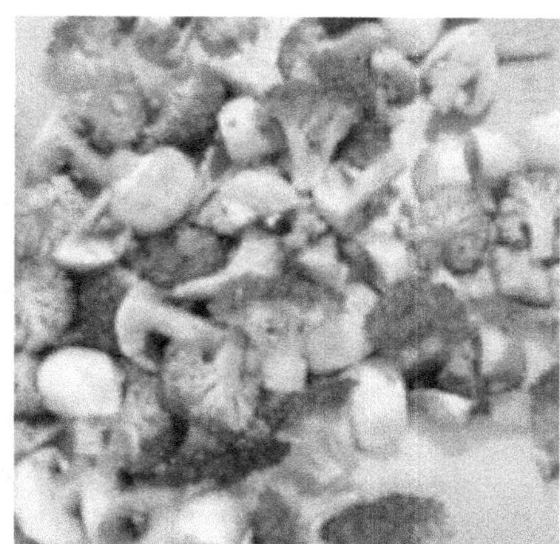

Mushroom & Broccoli Mix

Serves: 2
Prep time: 35 minutes

Ingredients

- 2 cups thinly sliced button mushrooms
- 4 cups broccoli
- 2 tablespoons minced garlic
- ½ teaspoon dried oregano
- 4 tablespoons grated Parmesan
- Salt and pepper to taste

Directions

1. The oven to be preheated to 400° F.
2. In a large bowl, combine mushrooms and broccoli. Add the olive oil and toss or stir to coat.
3. Season with salt, pepper, and oregano.
4. Transfer the broccoli and mushrooms to a baking dish. Bake 25 minutes.
5. Serve.

Nutritional Value (Amount per Serving)

Protein: 12.7 g
Carbs: 10.9 g
Fats: 3.5 g

DINNER RECIPE

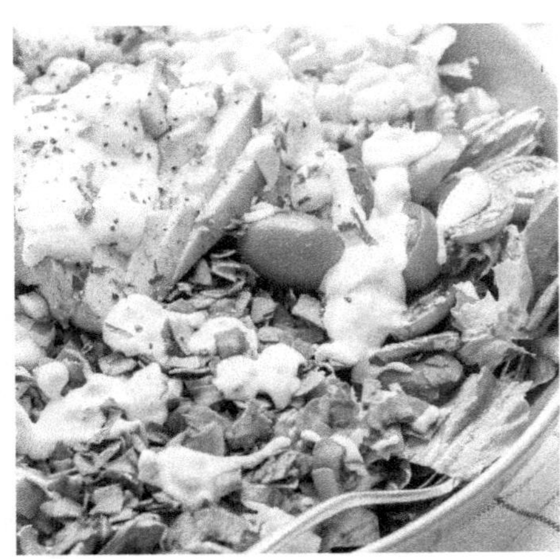

Easy and Healthy Spinach Cobb Salad

Serves: 2
Prep time: 10 minutes

Ingredients

- 2 boneless, skinless chicken breasts
- 4 slices bacon, cooked and crumbled
- 1 avocado, ripe and chopped
- 2 cups baby spinach, roughly chopped
- 1 cucumber, chopped
- 1 tomato, diced
- 2 hard-boiled eggs, chopped

Directions

1. Arrange the spinach on a serving platter.
2. Top the spinach with the remaining ingredients.
3. Serve and enjoy with ketogenic dressing.

Nutritional Value (Amount per Serving)

Protein: 31 g
Carbs: 6 g
Fat: 23 g

Day 13

Shopping list

- Tofu
- Non-dairy milk
- Onion
- Jalapeno
- Tomatoes
- Cilantro
- Potato
- Tortilla wraps
- Chili powder
- Salt and pepper
- Lemon juice
- Lime juice
- Clove garlic
- Avocado
- Black beans
- Cumin
- Chili powder
- Garlic powder
- Portobello mushroom caps
- Red bell pepper
- Orange bell pepper
- Salt and pepper
- Virgin olive oil
- Spinach
- Potatoes
- Spinach
- Parsley
- Carrots
- Vegetable broth

BREAKFAST RECIPE

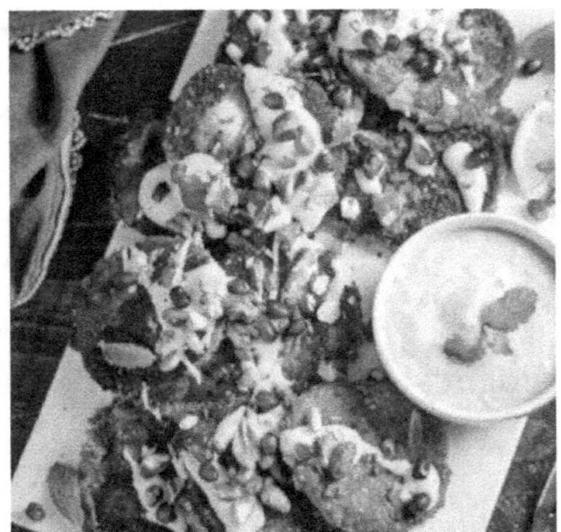

SUBTLE ROASTED EGGPLANT WITH FETA DIP

Serves: 12
Prep time: 40 minutes

Ingredients

- ¼ teaspoon cayenne pepper
- 2 tablespoons lemon juice
- 1 tablespoon finely chopped flat-leaf parsley
- ½ cup crumbled feta cheese
- 1 finely chopped small red bell pepper
- ¼ cup extra virgin olive oil
- 1 small chili pepper, seeded and minced
- 2 tablespoons chopped fresh basil
- 1 medium eggplant
- ¼ teaspoon salt
- Just a pinch of sugar

Directions

1. Preheat the broiler, positioning an oven rack about 6 inches below the heating element.
2. Line a baking pan with foil.
3. Gently poke holes all over the eggplant with a fork, and place on the pan.
4. Broil for about 18 minutes, turning the eggplant every 5 minutes.
5. Transfer the charred eggplant to a cutting board and let it cool.
6. In a medium-sized bowl, add the lemon juice.
7. Cut the eggplant in half lengthwise and scoop the flesh into the bowl.
8. Toss the flesh with the juice.
9. Add the oil and mash the mixture using a fork.
10. Stir in onion, feta, chili pepper, bell pepper, parsley, basil, salt and cayenne.
11. Mix well.
12. Season with sugar if desired.

Nutrition Value (Amount per Serving)

Protein: 2g
Carbs: 4g
Fats: 6g
Calories: 76

LUNCH RECIPE

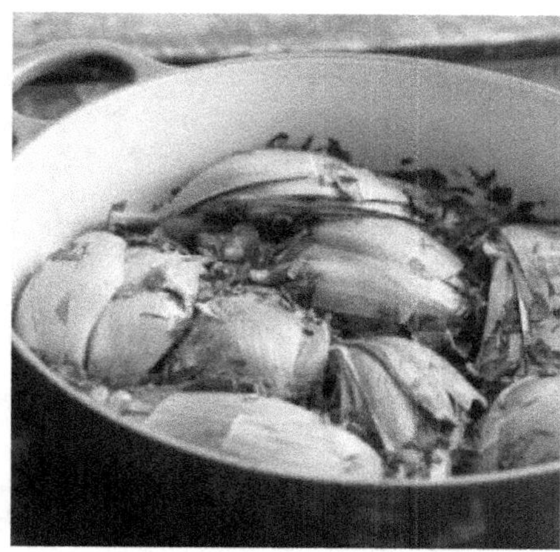

Slow-Cooker Sour Braised Artichokes

Serves: 4
Prep time: 2-4 hours

Ingredients

- 4 artichokes
- 4 tablespoons lemon juice
- 2 tablespoons melted coconut butter
- Salt and pepper to taste
- Fresh chopped thyme

Directions

1. Rinse artichokes and trim by removing leaves, layer by layer, until light yellow leaves are left.
2. Place the artichokes, lemon juice, melted coconut butter and salt in the slow cooker.
3. Cook until the artichokes are fork tender.
4. Transfer to platter. Garnish with chopped thyme. Serve.

Nutritional Value (Amount per Serving)

Protein: 4.3 g
Carbs: 14.5 g
Fat: 5.6 g

DINNER RECIPE

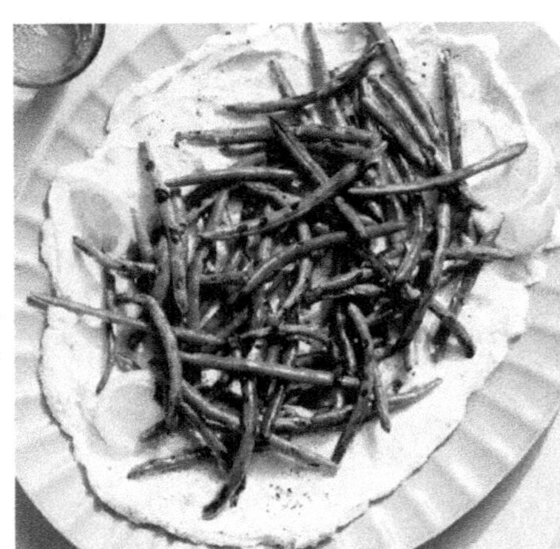

Lemon Green Beans & Caper Vinaigrette

Serves: 4
Prep time: 15 minutes

Ingredients

- 1 pound trimmed fresh green beans
- 3 tablespoons olive oil
- 2 tablespoons chopped capers
- Zest and juice from 1 lemon
- Salt and pepper to taste

Directions

1. Whisk together lemon juice, capers, oil, salt and pepper.
2. Boil and add 1 tablespoon of salt. Cook the green beans until tender, approximately 4-6 minutes.
3. Drain the beans and rinse in cold water.
4. Drizzle the caper vinaigrette over the beans and toss to coat. Transfer to plates. Serve.

Nutritional Value (Amount per Serving)

Protein: 1.8 g
Carbs: 8.7 g
Fat: 10.4 g

Day 14

Shopping list

- Tofu
- Non-dairy milk
- Onion
- Jalapeno
- Tomatoes
- Cilantro
- Potato
- Tortilla wraps
- Chili powder
- Salt and pepper
- Lemon juice
- Lime juice
- Clove garlic
- Avocado
- Black beans
- Cumin
- Chili powder
- Garlic powder
- Portobello mushroom caps
- Red bell pepper
- Orange bell pepper
- Salt and pepper
- Virgin olive oil
- Spinach
- Potatoes
- Spinach
- Parsley
- Carrots
- Vegetable broth

BREAKFAST RECIPE

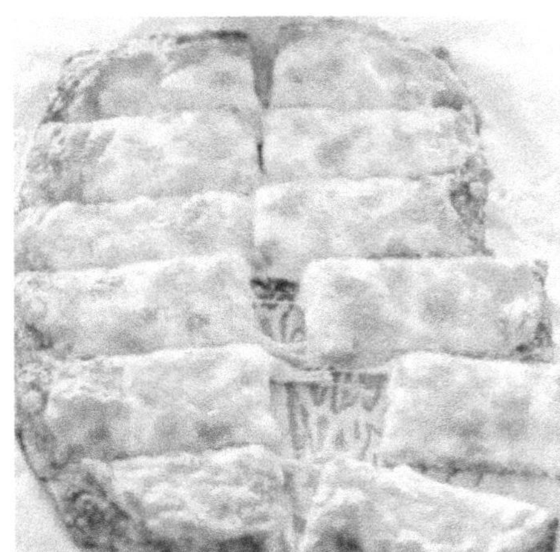

CAULIFLOWER MOZZARELLA STICKS

Serves: 6
Prep time: 50 minutes

Ingredients

- 1 medium cauliflower (to make 4 cups of cauliflower rice)
- 2 cups + 1 cup of mozzarella cheese
- 4 large eggs
- 4 cloves minced garlic
- 3 teaspoons fresh oregano
- Salt and pepper to taste
- Marinara sauce (for serving)

Directions

1. Preheat oven to 400☐F.
2. Rinse the cauliflower and pat dry. Cut into florets.
3. Place the florets in a food processor. Pulse until rice-like consistency.
4. Transfer the cauliflower rice to microwavable container. Cover and microwave 10 minutes.
5. Pour the cauliflower rice. Add 2 cups of mozzarella cheese, eggs, oregano, salt, pepper and garlic. Stir together.
6. Line two large baking trays with parchment paper. Spread the mixture in a single, even layer on the baking trays. Bake 25 minutes, until golden brown.
7. Remove the trays from the oven. Return to oven until cheese melts.
8. Remove from oven. Let rest 5 minutes. Slice into sticks.
9. Place marinara sauce in a small bowl for dipping. Serve.

Nutritional Value (Amount per Serving)

Protein: 21.7 g
Carbs: 6.7 g
Fat: 13.9 g

LUNCH RECIPE

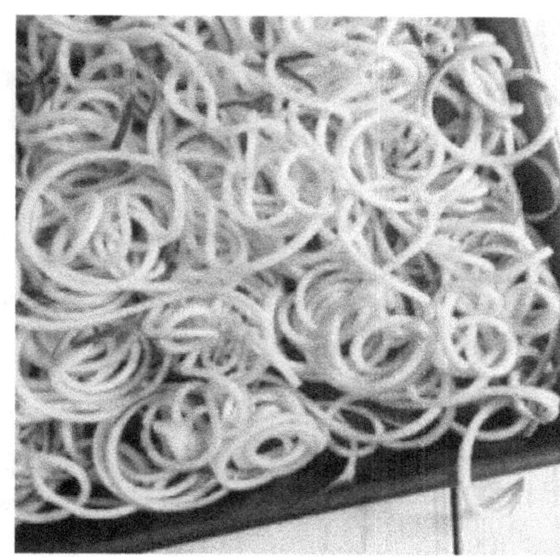

Basil Zucchini Noodles

Serves: 3
Prep time: 15 minutes

Ingredients

- 3 tablespoons chopped fresh basil
- 2 cups zucchini noodles
- 4 tablespoons extra virgin olive oil
- 4 cloves garlic, mashed
- 1 teaspoon red pepper flakes
- ½ bell red pepper, chopped
- Salt and pepper to taste

Directions

1. Turn zucchini into noodles.
2. Heat olive oil. Add garlic, red pepper flakes and red pepper.
3. Add zucchini noodles. Stir well. Cook 3 minutes.
4. Transfer the zucchini noodle mixture to a plate. Garnish with basil. Serve.

Nutritional Value (Amount per Serving)

Protein: 3.9 g
Carbs: 5.6 g
Fat: 15.6 g

DINNER RECIPE

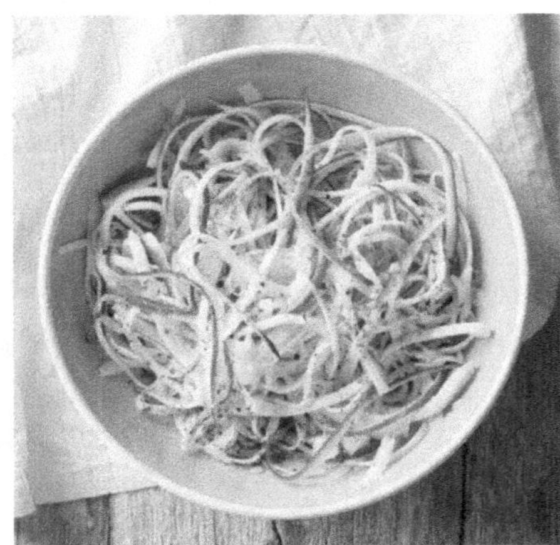

Ravishing Courgette Ribbon Salad

Serves: 4
Prep time: 15 minutes

Ingredients

- Juice of 1 lemon
- 2 tablespoons olive oil
- ½ a small package of chives, chopped
- ½ a small package of mint, chopped
- 300g courgettes
- Salt and pepper to taste

Directions

1. Add lemon juice, salt and pepper.
2. Whisk in olive oil and add the chopped herbs.
3. Pass the courgette through a spiralizer, making sure that the noodle attachment is placed so as to cut the courgette into spaghetti shape.
4. Tip the courgette ribbons into bowl.
5. Add dressing and toss well.
6. Serve!

Nutrition Value (Amount per Serving)

Protein: 29 g
Carbs: 65 g
Fats: 8 g

Day 15

Shopping list

- Tofu
- Non-dairy milk
- Onion
- Jalapeno
- Tomatoes
- Cilantro
- Potato
- Tortilla wraps
- Chili powder
- Salt and pepper
- Lemon juice
- Lime juice
- Clove garlic
- Avocado
- Black beans
- Cumin
- Chili powder
- Garlic powder
- Portobello mushroom caps
- Red bell pepper
- Orange bell pepper
- Salt and pepper
- Virgin olive oil
- Spinach
- Potatoes
- Spinach
- Parsley
- Carrots
- Vegetable broth

BREAKFAST RECIPE

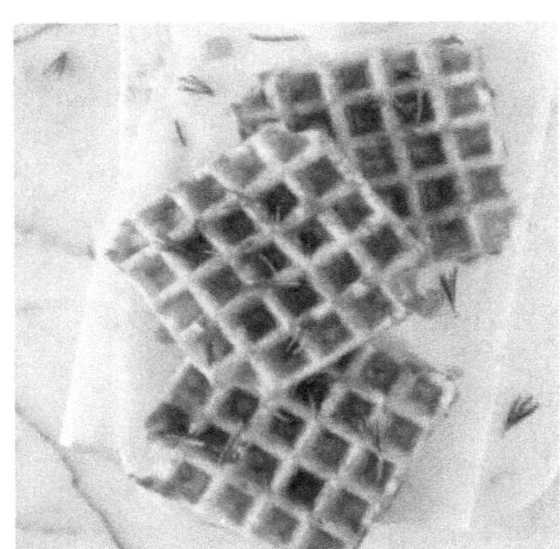

FLAXSEED SAVOURY WAFFLES

Serves: 6
Prep time: 15 minutes

Ingredients

- 5 large eggs
- 2 cups ground flaxseed
- 1 tablespoon baking powder (gluten-free)
- ½ teaspoon sea salt
- 1 cup water
- ½ cup melted coconut oil
- 1 tablespoon fresh herbs (sage, cilantro, parsley, basil)

Directions

1. Pre-heat waffle maker to medium heat.
2. Combine baking powder, salt, and flaxseed. Whisk thoroughly.
3. In a separate bowl, add eggs, oil and water. Using a whisk or handheld mixer, blend until fully combined. Pour the egg mixture in with the flaxseed mixture. Stir together. Let rest 5 minutes. Add the fresh herbs. Stir well.
4. Pour ¼ cup of mixture onto waffle maker. Cook 3 – 5 minutes.
5. Serve.

Nutritional Value (Amount per Serving)

Protein: 5.2 g
Carbs: 1.5 g
Fats: 16 g

LUNCH RECIPE

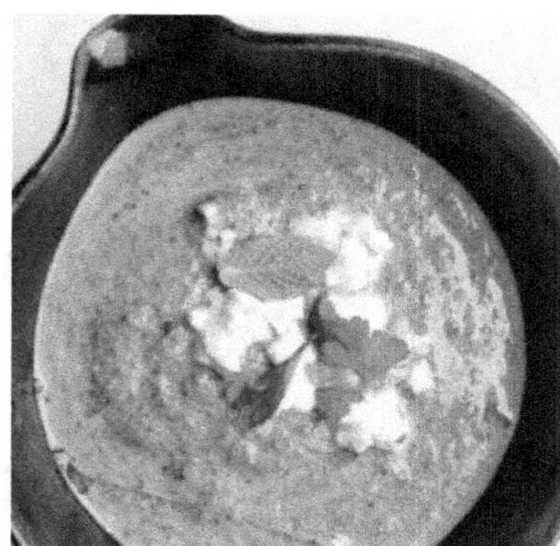

SPINACH PUREE AND SWISS CHARD

Serves: 8
Prep time: 25 minutes

Ingredients

- ½ pound swiss chard
- 1-pound baby spinach leaves
- 1 cup cauliflower florets
- 1 leek
- 4 tablespoons extra virgin olive oil
- 3 cups water
- ¼ cup cream cheese
- Salt and pepper to taste

Directions

1. Rinse the leek. Cut into thick slices.
2. Heat olive oil. Add the cauliflower and leek. Cook for 3 minutes.
3. Add spinach leaves, swiss chard, salt and pepper. Simmer 15 minutes.
4. Allow the vegetables to cool down, 10 minutes. Transfer to food processor. Blend until smooth.
5. Return the soup to the pan and put back on the heat. Stir in the cream cheese and water. Heat 5 minutes.
6. Pour into bowls. Serve.

Nutritional Value (Amount per Serving)

Protein: 3 g
Carbs: 8.7 g
Fat: 2.8 g

DINNER RECIPE

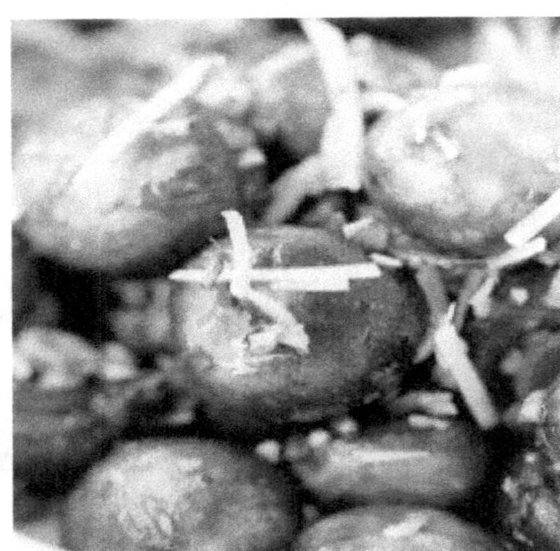

Mushrooms Roasted with Herbs & Parmesan

Serves: 6
Prep time: 35 minutes

Ingredients

- 1 pound Cremini mushrooms
- 1 can diced tomatoes
- 2 cups grated Parmesan cheese
- 2 tablespoons ghee
- 2 tablespoons mashed garlic

- 1 tablespoon fresh parsley
- 2 tablespoons fresh basil
- 1 tablespoon fresh thyme
- Salt and pepper to taste

Directions

1. The oven to be preheated to 400°F. Rinse the mushrooms, pat dry. Slice off stems.
2. In a large non-stick, oven-safe frying pan, melt the ghee.
3. Sauté the mushrooms for 5 minutes. Season with salt and pepper.
4. In a medium bowl, combine the herbs, tomatoes, salt and pepper. Stir mixture in with mushrooms. Sprinkle Parmesan cheese over top. Bake 25 minutes.
5. Remove from oven. Divide on plates. Serve.

Nutritional Value (Amount per Serving)

Protein: 14.8 g
Carbs: 5.3 g
Fat: 9.7 g

Day 16

Shopping list

- Tofu
- Non-dairy milk
- Onion
- Jalapeno
- Tomatoes
- Cilantro
- Potato
- Tortilla wraps
- Chili powder
- Salt and pepper
- Lemon juice
- Lime juice
- Clove garlic
- Avocado
- Black beans
- Cumin
- Chili powder
- Garlic powder
- Portobello mushroom caps
- Red bell pepper
- Orange bell pepper
- Salt and pepper
- Virgin olive oil
- Spinach
- Potatoes
- Spinach
- Parsley
- Carrots
- Vegetable broth

BREAKFAST RECIPE

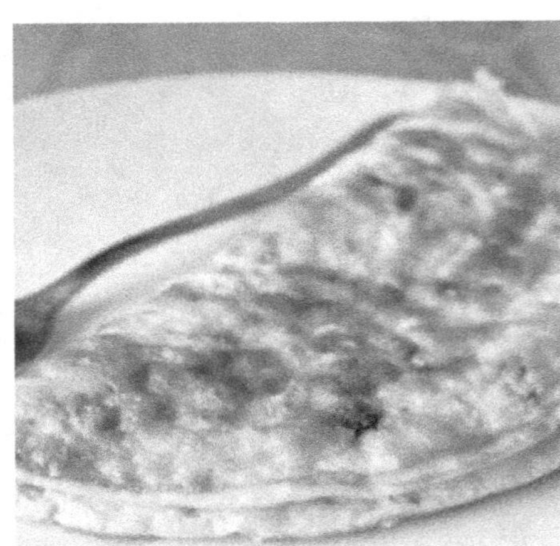

FETA MINTY OMELETTE

Serves: 2
Prep time: 15 minutes

Ingredients

- 3 large eggs
- 6 mint leaves
- 4 ounces' feta cheese
- Salt and pepper to taste
- Olive oil for frying

Directions

1. The oven to be preheated to 400□F.

2. In a medium bowl, combine eggs, feta cheese, mint leaves, salt and pepper. Whisk thoroughly.

3. In a non-stick, oven-safe frying pan, heat up some olive oil (a light layer drizzled over the bottom). Pour the egg mixture into the frying pan. Cook for 3 minutes.

4. Remove frying pan from stove and place in the oven. Cook 5 minutes.

5. Transfer omelette to a plate. Serve.

Nutrition Value (Amount per Serving)

Protein: 9.9 g
Carbs: 0.8 g
Fat: 7.6 g

LUNCH RECIPE

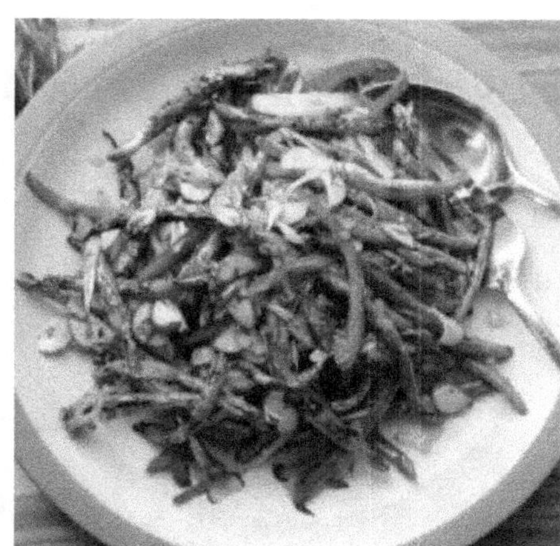

Pressure-Cooker Greens and Red-Hot Salad

Serves: 6
Prep time: 15 minutes

Ingredients

- 1½ pounds red cabbage, sliced into small wedges
- 1½ pounds Brussels sprouts, sliced into small wedges
- 3 medium beets, sliced into small wedges
- 8 cloves garlic, minced
- 3 tablespoons olive oil
- 1 tablespoon finely chopped fresh thyme

Directions

1. Place the vegetables and garlic in a pressure cooker.
2. Add the salt, pepper, thyme, and oil. Stir.
3. Set the cooker on Sauté. Cook for 15 minutes on high pressure.
4. Once ready, select natural release. Allow the pressure to go down naturally. (Approximately 15 - 20 minutes.)
5. Transfer vegetables to a platter. Serve.

Nutritional Value (Amount per Serving)

Protein: 6.5 g
Carbs: 13.4 g
Fat: 7.3 g

DINNER RECIPE

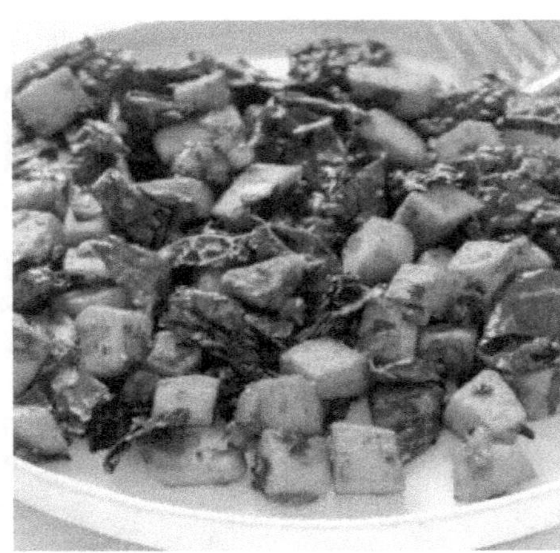

EGG WITH POWER GREENS AND SWEET POTATO CASSEROLE

Serves: 4
Prep time: 1 hour and 10 minutes

Ingredients

- 8 large eggs
- ½ teaspoon coconut oil
- 4 cups power greens (spinach, kale, arugula)
- 2 peeled sweet potatoes, diced
- 1 green onion, chopped
- ¼ cup coconut milk
- 1 teaspoon garlic powder
- ¼ teaspoon nutmeg
- Salt and pepper to taste
- Seasoning blend of your choice

Directions

1. Preheat oven to 400° F. Grease a casserole dish with coconut oil.
2. In a large bowl, whisk the eggs. Add the green onion, sweet potato, coconut milk, power greens and seasoning. Pour the egg mixture into the casserole.
3. Place dish in the oven. Bake 45 minutes.
4. Remove dish from the oven. Cover with foil. Bake for 15 more minutes.
5. Remove from oven. Cut into pieces and serve.

Nutritional Value (Amount per Serving)

Protein: 13.8 g
Carbs: 10.8 g
Fat: 11.9 g

Day 17

Shopping list

- Tofu
- Non-dairy milk
- Onion
- Jalapeno
- Tomatoes
- Cilantro
- Potato
- Tortilla wraps
- Chili powder
- Salt and pepper
- Lemon juice
- Lime juice
- Clove garlic
- Avocado
- Black beans
- Cumin
- Chili powder
- Garlic powder
- Portobello mushroom caps
- Red bell pepper
- Orange bell pepper
- Salt and pepper
- Virgin olive oil
- Spinach
- Potatoes
- Spinach
- Parsley
- Carrots
- Vegetable broth

BREAKFAST RECIPE

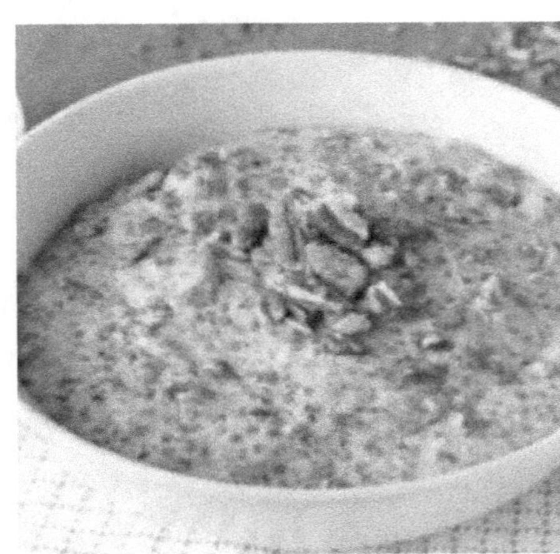

Flax Meal Cinnamon Porridge

Serves: 1
Prep time: 5 minutes

Ingredients

- 4 tablespoons soft cream cheese
- 4 tablespoons flax meal
- 1 cup water
- 1 cup sweetener
- Ground cinnamon to taste

Directions

1. Add all of the ingredients. Stir well.
2. Microwave for 2 minutes. Stir again. Top with fresh berries.
3. Serve.

Nutritional Value (Amount per Serving)

Protein: 3.4 g
Carbs: 6 g
Fat: 10.5 g

LUNCH RECIPE

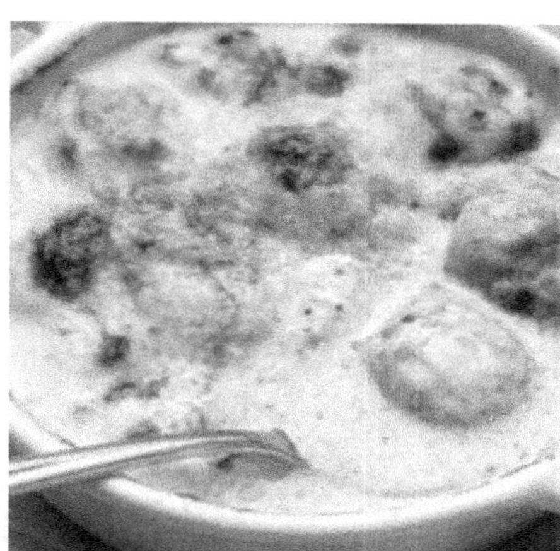

Creamy Cheesy Brussels Sprouts

Serves: 2
Prep time: 15 minutes

Ingredients

- 25 Brussels sprouts
- 4 cloves garlic, minced
- ¾ cup cream cheese
- 2 tablespoons extra virgin olive oil
- 2 teaspoons organic fresh lemon juice
- Salt and pepper to taste

Directions

1. Rinse the Brussels sprouts in cold water. Remove the stems.
2. Heat olive oil.
3. Add the minced garlic and Brussels sprouts to the pan. Sauté until tender.
4. Stir in the cream cheese and lemon juice.
5. Transfer to bowls. Serve.

Nutritional Value (Amount per Serving)

Protein: 11.7 g
Carbs: 18.5 g
Fat: 9.8 g

DINNER RECIPE

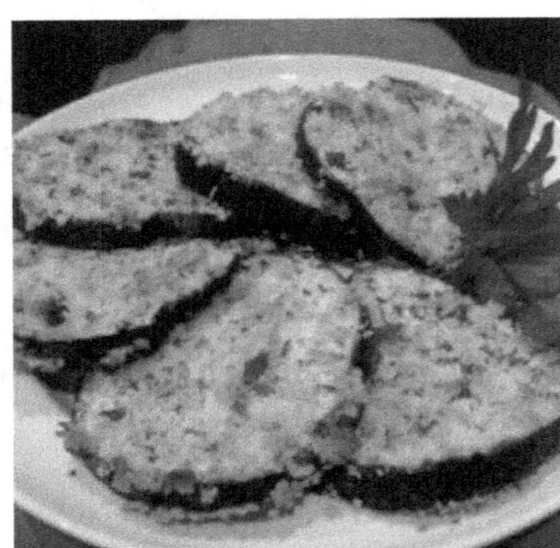

CHEESY FRIED EGGPLANT SLICES

Serves: 6
Prep time: 20 minutes

Ingredients

- 1 eggplant
- 1 large egg
- 1 cup almond flour
- 1 cup grated Parmesan cheese
- ½ cup coconut oil or butter
- Garlic powder
- Salt and pepper to taste

Directions

1. Rinse the eggplant and pat dry. Cut into slices, ½ inch thick. Arrange on a plate.

2. Sprinkle with salt. Let sit for 30 minutes.

3. Whisk the egg. Combine Parmesan cheese, garlic powder, almond flour, salt and pepper. Stir well.

4. Heat butter.

5. Fry until crispy and golden brown.

6. Place the cooked eggplant on a paper towel-lined plate to drain excess oil. Repeat with remaining eggplant slices.

7. Serve.

Nutritional Value (Amount per Serving)

Protein: 13.2 g
Carbs: 7.9 g
Fat: 33 g

Day 18

Shopping list

- Tofu
- Non-dairy milk
- Onion
- Jalapeno
- Tomatoes
- Cilantro
- Potato
- Tortilla wraps
- Chili powder
- Salt and pepper
- Lemon juice
- Lime juice
- Clove garlic
- Avocado
- Black beans
- Cumin
- Chili powder
- Garlic powder
- Portobello mushroom caps
- Red bell pepper
- Orange bell pepper
- Salt and pepper
- Virgin olive oil
- Spinach
- Potatoes
- Spinach
- Parsley
- Carrots
- Vegetable broth

BREAKFAST RECIPE

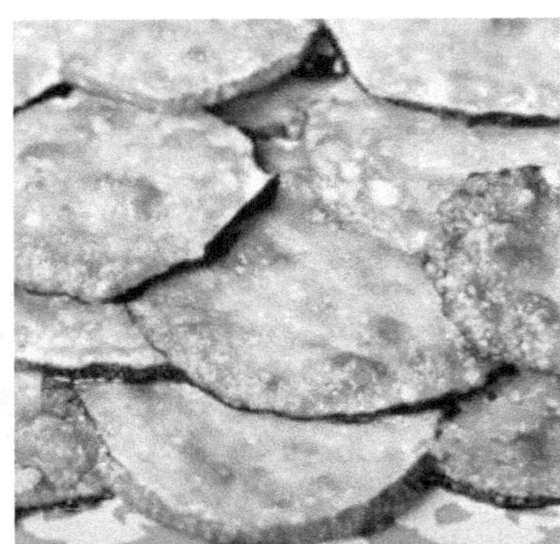

Baked Zucchini Parmigianino

Serves: 6
Prep Time: 40 minutes

Ingredients

- 3 large eggs
- 1 cup almond flour
- 1 cup ground almonds
- 2 zucchinis, thinly sliced
- 1 cup Parmigiano-Reggiano cheese, grated
- 1 teaspoon dried oregano
- Salt and pepper to taste

Directions

1. The oven to be preheated to 400□F.
2. In a large bowl combine the oregano and Parmigiano-Reggiano cheese. Season with salt and pepper to taste. Set aside.
3. Pour the almond flour into a separate bowl.
4. In a third bowl, whisk the eggs together. Season with salt and pepper to taste.
5. Dip sliced zucchini in flour, then in the egg mixture, then in the almond flour.
6. Bake 30 minutes. Serve.

Nutritional Value (Amount per Serving)

Protein: 14.1 g
Carbs: 13.8 g
Fat: 17.5 g

LUNCH RECIPE

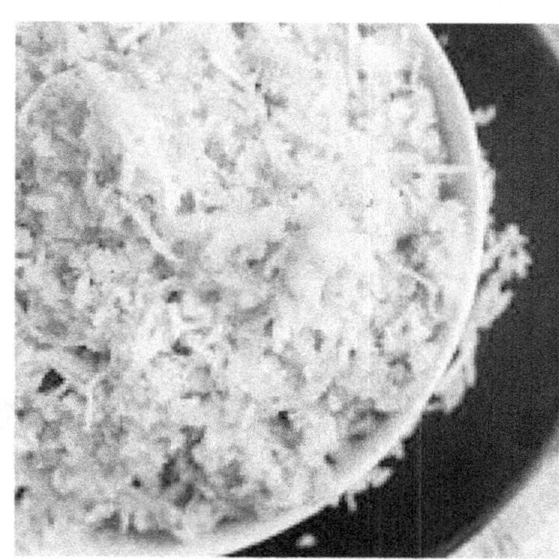

CAULIFLOWER COCONUT RICE

Serves: 3
Prep Time: 20 minutes

Ingredients

- 3 cups cauliflower rice
- ½ tsp onion powder
- 1 tsp chili paste
- 2/3 cup coconut milk
- Salt

Directions

1. Add all ingredients to the pan and heat over medium-low heat. Stir to combine.

2. Cook for 10 minutes. Stir after every 2 minutes.

3. Remove lid and cook until excess liquid absorbed.

4. Serve and enjoy.

Nutritional Value (Amount per Serving)

Protein: 3.4 g
Carbs: 9.2 g
Fat: 13.1 g
Sugar: 4.8 g
Calories: 155
Cholesterol: 1 mg

DINNER RECIPE

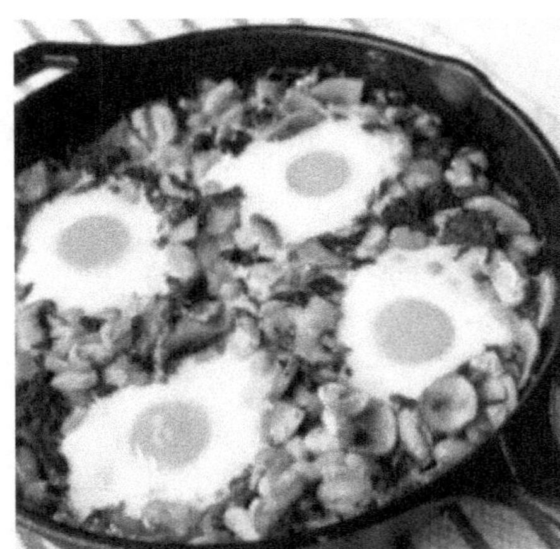

Broiled Eggs

Serves: 2
Prep Time: 20 minutes

Ingredients

- 4 large eggs
- 6 tablespoons heavy cream
- 1 tablespoon extra-virgin olive oil
- 1 tablespoon Parmesan cheese, plus extra for serving
- ¼ cup button mushrooms, sliced
- ¼ cup baby spinach
- 1 pinch red pepper flakes
- Salt and pepper to taste

Directions

1. Preheat broiler to 400□F. Rinse mushrooms, pat dry.
2. In a large non-stick, oven-safe frying pan, heat the oil over medium heat. Fry the eggs on one side for 3 minutes. Remove to a plate and set aside.
3. Pour half the heavy cream in the pan. Add the mushrooms. Simmer for 3 minutes.
4. Stir in the remaining heavy cream. Add the Parmesan cheese. Stir well.
5. Place under broiler for 3 minutes.
6. Pull the pan out of the oven. Add the spinach leaves and red pepper flakes. Stir well.
7. Return the eggs to the pan. Return the pan to the broiler for 2-3 minutes.
8. Remove the pan from the oven. Sprinkle more Parmesan cheese over top.
9. Garnish with fresh spinach leaves. Serve.

Nutritional Value (Amount per Serving)

Protein: 8.5 g
Carbs: 2.8 g
Fat: 20.9 g

Day 19

Shopping list

- Tofu
- Non-dairy milk
- Onion
- Jalapeno
- Tomatoes
- Cilantro
- Potato
- Tortilla wraps
- Chili powder
- Salt and pepper
- Lemon juice
- Lime juice
- Clove garlic
- Avocado
- Black beans
- Cumin
- Chili powder
- Garlic powder
- Portobello mushroom caps
- Red bell pepper
- Orange bell pepper
- Salt and pepper
- Virgin olive oil
- Spinach
- Potatoes
- Spinach
- Parsley
- Carrots
- Vegetable broth

BREAKFAST RECIPE

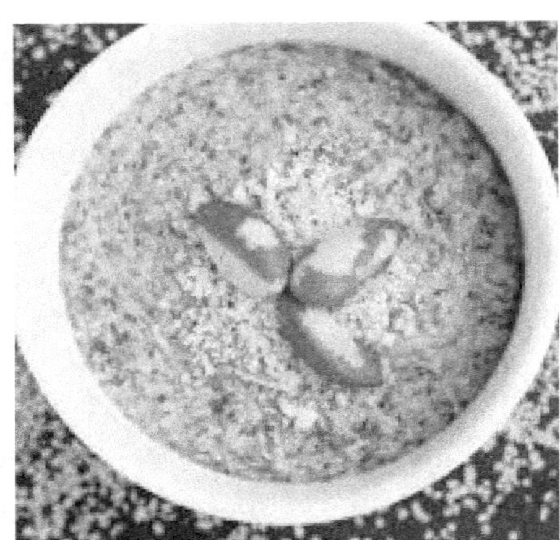

ALMOND HEMP HEART PORRIDGE

Serves: 2
Prep Time: 10 minutes

Ingredients:

- ¼ cup almond flour
- ½ tsp cinnamon
- ¾ tsp vanilla extract
- 5 drops stevia
- 1 tbsp chia seeds
- 2 tbsp ground flax seed
- ½ cup hemp hearts
- 1 cup unsweetened coconut milk

Directions:

1. Add all ingredients except almond flour to a saucepan. Stir to combine.
2. Heat over medium heat until just starts to lightly boil.
3. Once start bubbling then stir well and cook for 1 minute more.
4. Remove from heat and stir in almond flour.

Nutritional Value (Amount per Serving)

Protein: 16.2 g
Carbs: 9.2 g
Fat: 24.4 g
Sugar: 1.8 g
Calories: 329
Cholesterol: 0 mg

LUNCH RECIPE

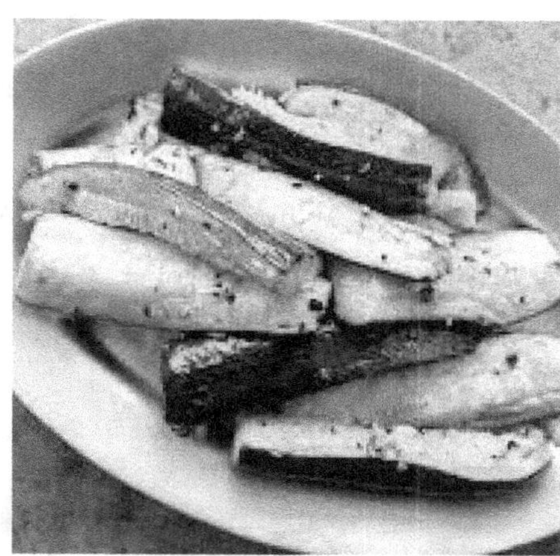

Garlic Zucchini Squash

Serves: 4
Prep Time: 20 minutes

Ingredients

- 1 small squash, sliced
- 2 tbsp fresh basil, chopped
- 2 tbsp olive oil
- 1 garlic clove, chopped
- 1 large onion, sliced
- 2 fresh tomatoes, cut into wedges
- 1 small zucchini, sliced
- Pepper
- Salt

Directions

1. Heat olive oil.
2. Add onion, squash, zucchini, and garlic and sauté until lightly brown.
3. Add basil and tomatoes and cook for 5 minutes. Season with pepper and salt.
4. Simmer over low heat until squash is tender.
5. Stir well and serve.

Nutritional Value (Amount per Serving)

Protein: 1.4 g
Carbs: 8.2 g
Fat: 7.2 g
Sugar: 4.4 g
Calories: 97;
Cholesterol: 0 mg;

DINNER RECIPE

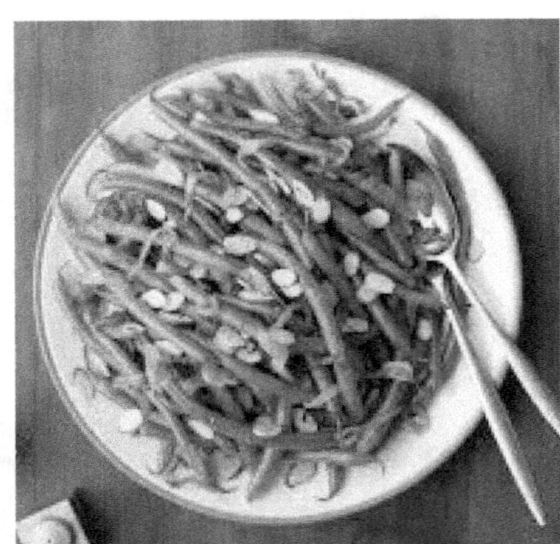

ALMOND GREEN BEANS

Serves: 4
Prep Time: 20 minutes

Ingredients:

- 1 lb fresh green beans, trimmed
- 1/3 cup almonds, sliced
- 4 garlic cloves, sliced
- 2 tbsp olive oil
- 1 tbsp lemon juice
- ½ tsp sea salt

Directions:

1. Add green beans, salt, and lemon juice in a mixing bowl. Toss well and set aside.
2. Heat oil in a pan over medium heat.
3. Add sliced almonds and sauté until lightly browned.
4. Add garlic and sauté for 30 seconds.
5. Pour almond mixture over green beans and toss well.
6. Stir well and serve immediately.

Nutritional Value (Amount per Serving)

Protein: 4 g
Carbs: 10.9 g
Fat: 11.2 g
Sugar: 2 g
Calories: 146
Cholesterol: 0 mg;

Day 20

Shopping list

- Tofu
- Non-dairy milk
- Onion
- Jalapeno
- Tomatoes
- Cilantro
- Potato
- Tortilla wraps
- Chili powder
- Salt and pepper
- Lemon juice
- Lime juice
- Clove garlic
- Avocado
- Black beans
- Cumin
- Chili powder
- Garlic powder
- Portobello mushroom caps
- Red bell pepper
- Orange bell pepper
- Salt and pepper
- Virgin olive oil
- Spinach
- Potatoes
- Spinach
- Parsley
- Carrots
- Vegetable broth

BREAKFAST RECIPE

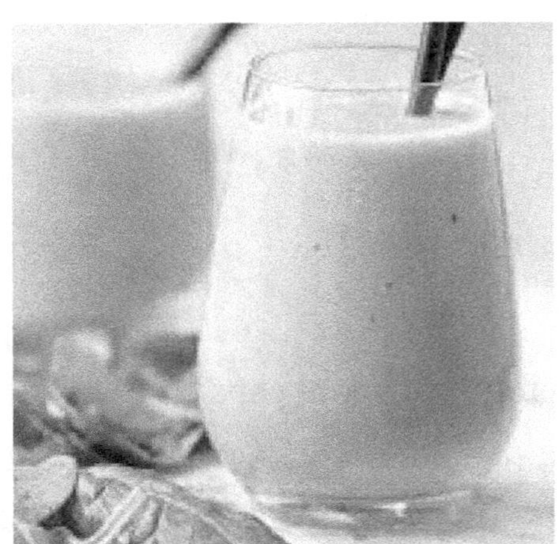

Healthy Spinach Green Smoothie

Serves: 1
Prep Time: 5 minutes

Ingredients

- 1 cup ice cube
- 2/3 cup water
- ½ cup unsweetened almond milk
- 5 drops liquid stevia
- ½ tsp matcha powder
- 1 tsp vanilla extract
- 1 tbsp MCT oil
- ½ avocado
- 2/3 cup spinach

Directions

1. Blend until smooth and creamy then serve.

Nutritional Value (Amount per Serving)

Protein: 1.6 g
Carbs: 3.8 g
Fat: 18.3 g
Sugar: 0.6 g
Calories: 167
Cholesterol: 0 mg

LUNCH RECIPE

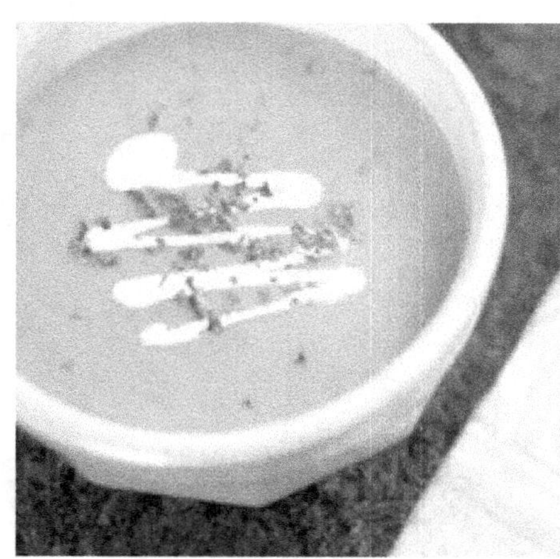

CREAMY SQUASH SOUP

Serves: 8
Prep Time: 35 minutes

Ingredients

- 3 cups butternut squash, chopped
- 1 ½ cups unsweetened coconut milk
- 1 tbsp coconut oil
- 1 tsp dried onion flakes
- 1 tbsp curry powder
- 4 cups water
- 1 garlic clove
- 1 tsp kosher salt

Directions

1. Add squash, coconut oil, onion flakes, curry powder, water, garlic, and salt into a large saucepan. Bring to boil over high heat.
2. Simmer for 20 minutes.
3. Puree the soup using a blender until smooth. Cook for 2 minutes.
4. Stir well and serve hot.

Nutritional Value (Amount per Serving)

Protein: 1.7 g
Carbs: 9.4 g
Fat: 12.6 g
Sugar: 2.8 g
Calories: 146
Cholesterol: 0 mg

DINNER RECIPE

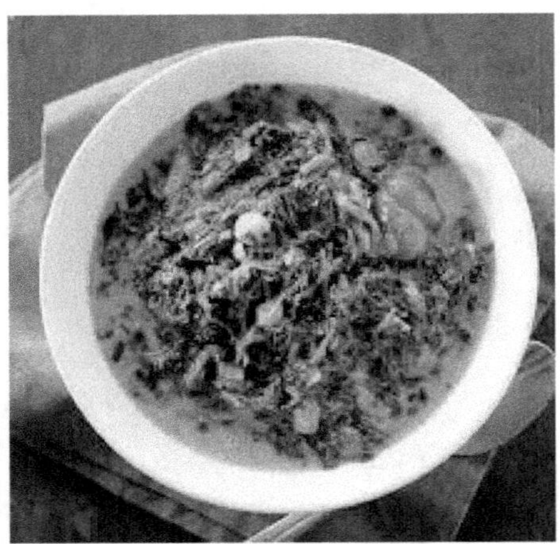

SPINACH WITH COCONUT MILK

Serves: 6
Prep Time: 25 minutes

Ingredients

- 16 oz spinach
- 2 tsp curry powder
- 13.5 oz coconut milk
- 1 tsp lemon zest
- ½ tsp salt

Directions

1. Add spinach in pan and heat over medium heat. Once it is hot then add curry paste and few tablespoons of coconut milk. Stir well.

2. Add remaining coconut milk, lemon zest, and salt and cook until thickened.

3. Serve and enjoy.

Nutritional Value (Amount per Serving)

Protein: 3.7 g
Carbs: 6.7 g
Fat: 15.6 g
Sugar: 2.5 g
Calories: 167
Cholesterol: 0 mg

Day 21

Shopping list

- Tofu
- Non-dairy milk
- Onion
- Jalapeno
- Tomatoes
- Cilantro
- Potato
- Tortilla wraps
- Chili powder
- Salt and pepper
- Lemon juice
- Lime juice
- Clove garlic
- Avocado
- Black beans
- Cumin
- Chili powder
- Garlic powder
- Portobello mushroom caps
- Red bell pepper
- Orange bell pepper
- Salt and pepper
- Virgin olive oil
- Spinach
- Potatoes
- Spinach
- Parsley
- Carrots
- Vegetable broth

BREAKFAST RECIPE

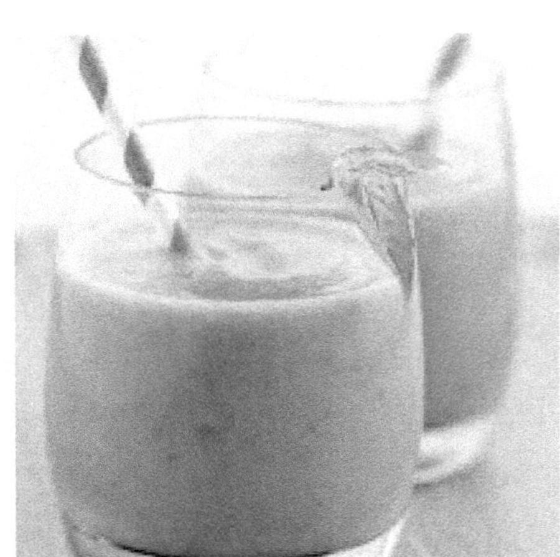

APPLE AVOCADO COCONUT SMOOTHIE

Serves: 2
Prep Time: 5 minutes

Ingredients

- 1 tsp coconut oil
- 1 tbsp collagen powder
- 1 tbsp fresh lime juice
- ½ cup unsweetened coconut milk
- ¼ apple, slice
- 1 avocado

Directions

1. Blend until smooth and creamy.
2. Serve and enjoy.

Nutritional Value (Amount per Serving)

Protein: 2 g
Carbs: 13.6 g
Fat: 23.9 g
Sugar: 3.4 g
Cholesterol: 0 mg

LUNCH RECIPE

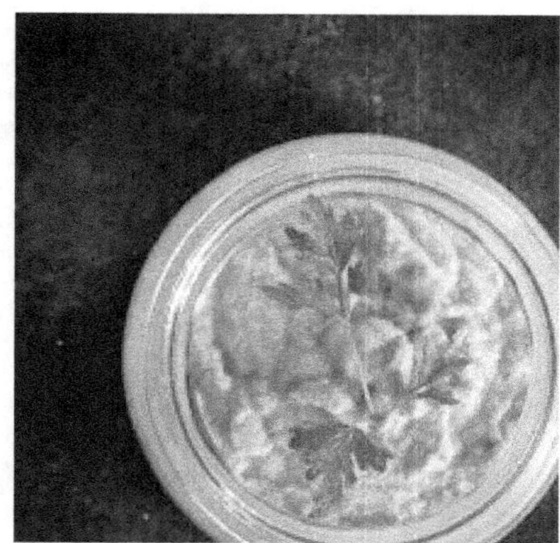

Asparagus Mash

Serves: 2
Prep Time: 20 minutes

Ingredients

- 10 asparagus shoots, chopped
- 1 tsp lemon juice
- 2 tbsp fresh parsley
- 2 tbsp coconut cream
- 1 small onion, diced
- 1 tbsp coconut oil
- Pepper
- Salt

Directions

1. Sauté onion in coconut oil until onion is softened.
2. Blanch chopped asparagus in hot water for 2 minutes and drain immediately.
3. Add sautéed onion, lemon juice, parsley, coconut cream, asparagus, pepper, and salt and blend until smooth.
4. Serve warm and enjoy.

Nutritional Value (Amount per Serving)

Protein: 2.6 g
Carbs: 7.5 g
Fat: 10.6 g
Sugar: 3.6 g
Calories: 125
Cholesterol: 0 mg

DINNER RECIPE

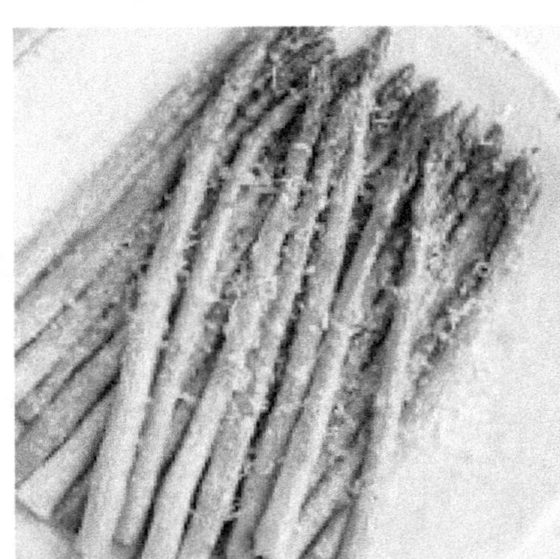

BAKED ASPARAGUS

Serves: 4
Prep Time: 25 minutes

Ingredients

- 40 asparagus spears
- 2 tbsp vegetable seasoning
- 2 tbsp garlic powder
- 2 tbsp salt

Directions

1. The oven to be preheated to 450 F/ 232 C.
2. Arrange all asparagus spears on baking tray and season with vegetable seasoning, garlic powder, and salt.
3. Bake for 20 minutes.
4. Serve warm and enjoy.

Nutritional Value (Amount per Serving)

Protein: 6.7 g
Carbs: 13.5 g
Fat: 0.9 g
Sugar: 5.5 g
Calories: 75
Cholesterol: 0 mg

Day 22

Shopping list

- Tofu
- Non-dairy milk
- Onion
- Jalapeno
- Tomatoes
- Cilantro
- Potato
- Tortilla wraps
- Chili powder
- Salt and pepper
- Lemon juice
- Lime juice
- Clove garlic
- Avocado
- Black beans
- Cumin
- Chili powder
- Garlic powder
- Portobello mushroom caps
- Red bell pepper
- Orange bell pepper
- Salt and pepper
- Virgin olive oil
- Spinach
- Potatoes
- Spinach
- Parsley
- Carrots
- Vegetable broth

BREAKFAST RECIPE

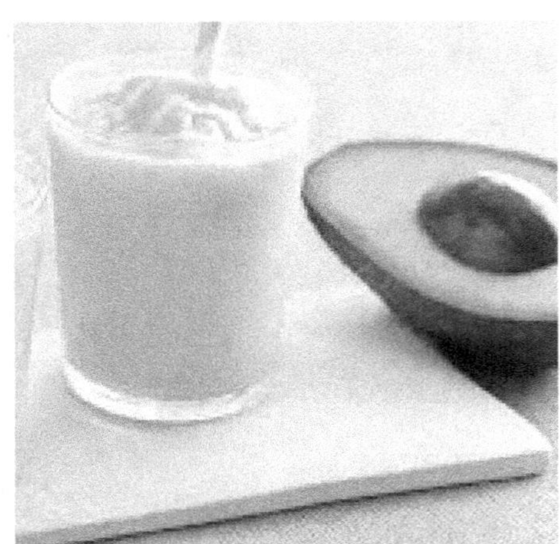

AVOCADO BREAKFAST SMOOTHIE

Serves: 2
Prep Time: 5 minutes

Ingredients

- 5 drops liquid stevia
- ¼ cup ice cubes
- ½ avocado
- 1 tsp vanilla extract
- 1 cup unsweetened coconut milk

Directions

1. Blend until smooth and creamy.
2. Serve immediately and enjoy.

Nutritional Value (Amount per Serving)

Protein: 1 g
Carbs: 5.6 g
Fat: 11.8 g
Sugar: 0.5 g
Calories: 131
Cholesterol: 0 mg

LUNCH RECIPE

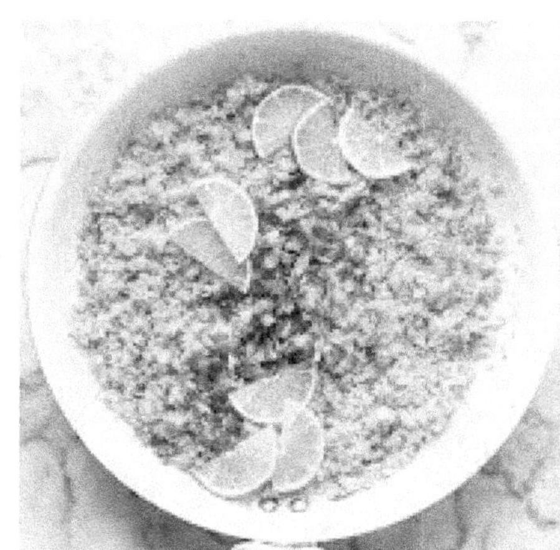

Mexican Cauliflower Rice

Serves: 4
Prep Time: 25 minutes

Ingredients

- 1 medium cauliflower head, cut into florets
- ½ cup tomato sauce
- ¼ tsp black pepper
- 1 tsp chili powder
- 2 garlic cloves, minced
- ½ medium onion, diced
- 1 tbsp coconut oil
- ½ tsp sea salt

Directions

1. Add cauliflower florets into the food processor and process until it looks like rice.
2. Heat oil in a pan over medium-high heat.
3. Add onion to the pan and sauté for 5 minutes or until softened.
4. Add garlic and cook for 1 minute.
5. Add cauliflower rice, chili powder, pepper, and salt. Stir well.
6. Cook for 5 minutes.
7. Stir well and serve warm.

Nutritional Value (Amount per Serving)

Protein: 3.6 g
Carbs: 11.5 g
Fat: 3.7g
Sugar: 5.4 g
Calories: 83
Cholesterol: 0 mg;

DINNER RECIPE

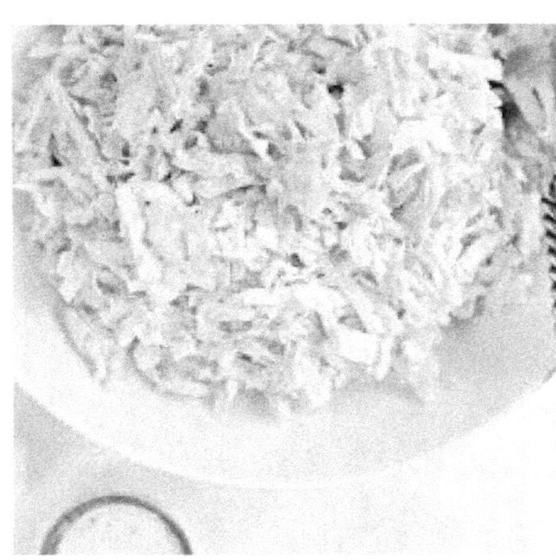

Classic Cabbage Slaw

Serves: 3
Prep Time: 20 minutes

Ingredients

- 4 cups green cabbage, shredded
- 2 garlic cloves
- 1 tbsp sesame oil
- 2 tbsp tamari
- 1 tsp vinegar
- 1 tsp chili paste
- ½ cup macadamia nuts, chopped

Directions

1. Toss shredded green cabbage in a pan with chili paste, sesame oil, vinegar, and tamari on medium-low heat.
2. Add garlic and cook for 5 minutes or until cabbage is softened.
3. Stir everything well. Add macadamia nuts and cook for 5 minutes.
4. Stir well and serve.

Nutritional Value (Amount per Serving)

Protein: 4.5 g
Carbs: 10.5 g
Fat: 21.8 g
Sugar: 4.7 g
Calories: 240
Cholesterol: 1 mg

Day 23

Shopping list

- Tofu
- Non-dairy milk
- Onion
- Jalapeno
- Tomatoes
- Cilantro
- Potato
- Tortilla wraps
- Chili powder
- Salt and pepper
- Lemon juice
- Lime juice
- Clove garlic
- Avocado
- Black beans
- Cumin
- Chili powder
- Garlic powder
- Portobello mushroom caps
- Red bell pepper
- Orange bell pepper
- Salt and pepper
- Virgin olive oil
- Spinach
- Potatoes
- Spinach
- Parsley
- Carrots
- Vegetable broth

BREAKFAST RECIPE

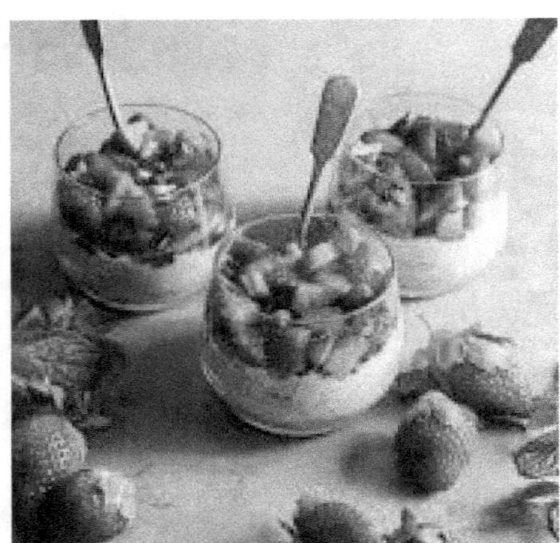

STRAWBERRY CHIA MATCHA PUDDING

Serves: 1
Prep Time: 10 minutes

Ingredients

- 5 drops liquid stevia
- 2 strawberries, diced
- 1 ½ tbsp chia seeds
- ¾ cup unsweetened coconut milk
- ½ tsp matcha powder

Directions

1. Add all ingredients except strawberries into the glass jar and mix well.
2. Close jar with lid and place in refrigerator for 4 hours.
3. Add strawberries into the pudding and mix well.
4. Serve and enjoy.

Nutritional Value (Amount per Serving)

Protein: 2.5 g
Carbs: 5.6 g
Fat: 6.5 g
Sugar: 1.2 g
Calories: 93
Cholesterol: 0 mg

LUNCH RECIPE

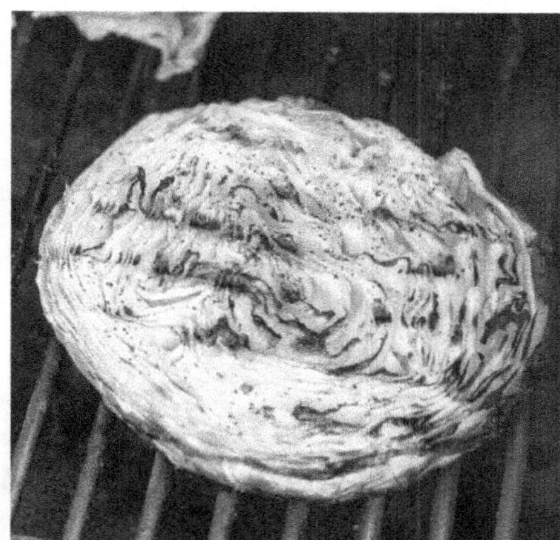

DELICIOUS CABBAGE STEAKS

Serves: 6
Prep Time: 1 hour and 20 minutes

Ingredients

- 1 medium cabbage head, slice 1" thick
- 2 tbsp olive oil
- 1 tbsp garlic, minced
- Pepper
- Salt

Directions

1. Mix together garlic and olive oil.
2. Brush garlic and olive oil mixture onto both sides of sliced cabbage.
3. Season cabbage slices with pepper and salt.
4. Place cabbage slices onto a baking tray and bake at 350 F/ 180 C for 1 hour. Turn after 30 minutes.
5. Serve and enjoy.

Nutritional Value (Amount per Serving)

Protein: 1.6 g
Carbs: 7.4 g
Fat: 4.8 g
Sugar: 3.8 g
Calories: 72
Cholesterol: 0 mg

DINNER RECIPE

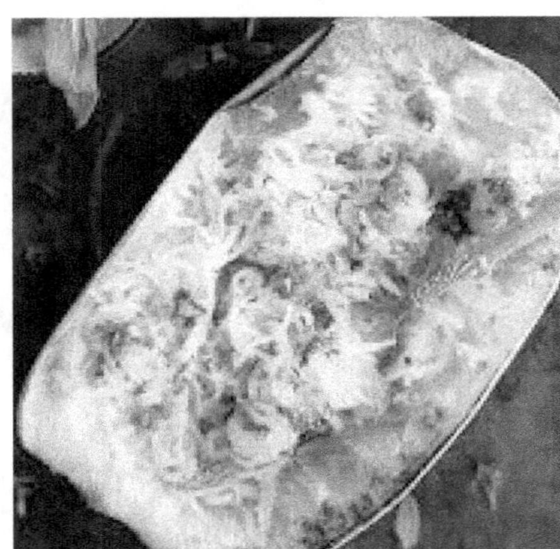

Herb Spaghetti Squash

Serves: 4
Prep Time: 30 minutes

Ingredients

- 4 cups spaghetti squash, cooked
- ½ tsp pepper
- ½ tsp sage
- 1 tsp dried parsley
- 1 tsp dried thyme
- 1 tsp dried rosemary
- 1 tsp garlic powder
- 2 tbsp olive oil
- 1 tsp salt

Directions

1. The oven to be preheated to 350 F/ 180 C.
2. Mix well to combine.
3. Transfer bowl mixture to the oven safe dish and cook in preheated oven for 15 minutes.
4. Stir well and serve.

Nutritional Value (Amount per Serving)

Protein: 0.9 g
Carbs: 8.1 g
Fat: 7.7 g
Sugar: 0.2 g
Calories: 96
Cholesterol: 0 mg

Day 24

Shopping list

- Tofu
- Non-dairy milk
- Onion
- Jalapeno
- Tomatoes
- Cilantro
- Potato
- Tortilla wraps
- Chili powder
- Salt and pepper
- Lemon juice
- Lime juice
- Clove garlic
- Avocado
- Black beans
- Cumin
- Chili powder
- Garlic powder
- Portobello mushroom caps
- Red bell pepper
- Orange bell pepper
- Salt and pepper
- Virgin olive oil
- Spinach
- Potatoes
- Spinach
- Parsley
- Carrots
- Vegetable broth

BREAKFAST RECIPE

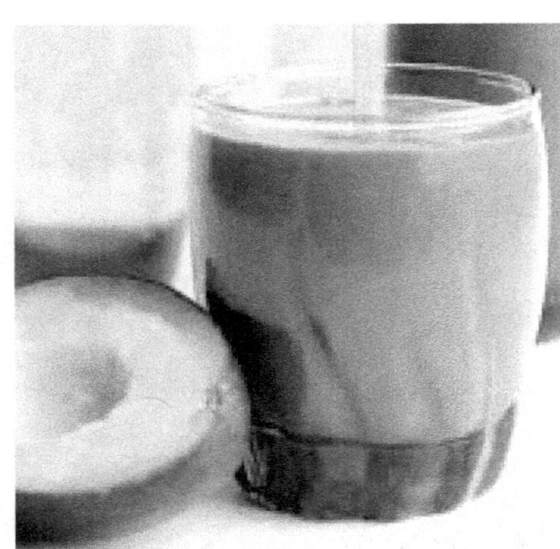

Avocado Chocó Cinnamon Smoothie

Serves: 1
Prep Time: 5 minutes

Ingredients

- ½ tsp coconut oil
- 5 drops liquid stevia
- ¼ tsp vanilla extract
- 1 tsp ground cinnamon
- 2 tsp unsweetened cocoa powder
- ½ avocado
- ¾ cup unsweetened coconut milk

Directions

1. Add all ingredients blend until smooth and creamy.
2. Serve immediately and enjoy.

Nutritional Value (Amount per Serving)

Protein: 1.2 g
Carbs: 5.1 g
Fat: 8.3 g
Sugar: 0.2 g
Calories: 95
Cholesterol: 0 mg

LUNCH RECIPE

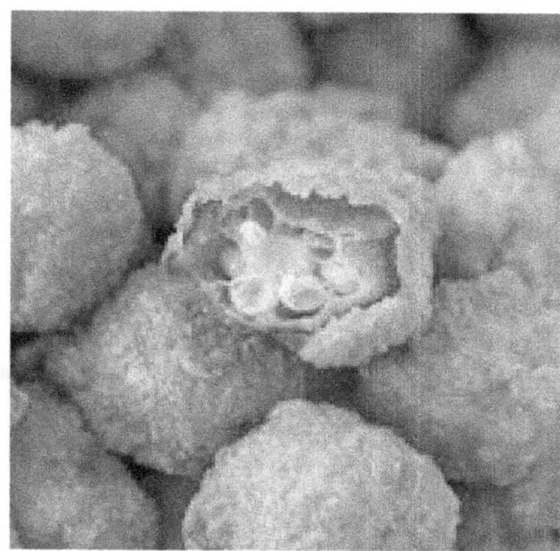

FRIED OKRA

Serves: 4
Prep Time: 20 minutes

Ingredients

- 1 lb fresh okra, cut into ¼" slices
- 1/3 cup almond meal
- Pepper
- Salt
- Oil for frying

Directions

1. Heat oil.
2. In a bowl, mix together sliced okra, almond meal, pepper, and salt until well coated.
3. Once the oil is hot then add okra to the hot oil and cook until lightly browned.
4. Remove fried okra from pan and allow to drain on paper towels.
5. Serve and enjoy.

Nutritional Value (Amount per Serving)

Protein: 3.9 g
Carbs: 10.2 g
Fat: 4.2 g
Sugar: 10.2 g
Calories: 91
Cholesterol: 0 mg

DINNER RECIPE

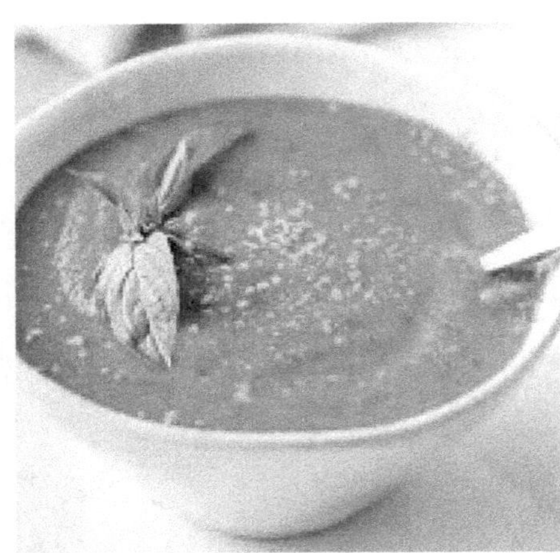

Basil Tomato Soup

Serves: 6
Prep Time: 20 minutes

Ingredients

- 28 oz can tomatoes
- ¼ cup basil pesto
- ¼ tsp dried basil leaves
- 1 tsp apple cider vinegar
- 2 tbsp erythritol
- ¼ tsp garlic powder
- ½ tsp onion powder
- 2 cups water
- 1 ½ tsp kosher salt

Directions

1. Add tomatoes, garlic powder, onion powder, water, and salt in a saucepan.
2. Bring to boil over medium heat. Reduce heat and simmer for 2 minutes.
3. Heat and blend until smooth.
4. Stir in pesto, dried basil, vinegar, and erythritol.
5. Stir well and serve warm.

Nutritional Value (Amount per Serving)

Protein: 1.3 g
Carbs: 12.2 g
Fat: 0 g
Sugar: 9.6 g
Calories: 30
Cholesterol: 0 mg

Day 25

Shopping list

- Tofu
- Non-dairy milk
- Onion
- Jalapeno
- Tomatoes
- Cilantro
- Potato
- Tortilla wraps
- Chili powder
- Salt and pepper
- Lemon juice
- Lime juice
- Clove garlic
- Avocado
- Black beans
- Cumin
- Chili powder
- Garlic powder
- Portobello mushroom caps
- Red bell pepper
- Orange bell pepper
- Salt and pepper
- Virgin olive oil
- Spinach
- Potatoes
- Spinach
- Parsley
- Carrots
- Vegetable broth

BREAKFAST RECIPE

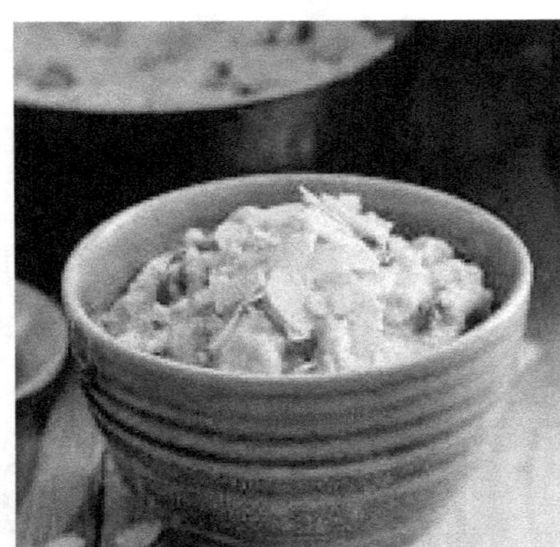

ALMOND COCONUT PORRIDGE

Serves: 2
Prep Time: 10 minutes

Ingredients

- ¾ cup unsweetened almond milk
- ½ tsp vanilla extract
- 1 ½ tbsp ground flaxseed
- 3 tbsp ground almonds
- 6 tbsp unsweetened shredded coconut
- Pinch of sea salt

Directions

1. Add almond milk in microwave safe bowl and microwave for 2 minutes.
2. Add remaining ingredients and stir well and cook for 1 minute.
3. Top with fresh berries and serve.

Nutritional Value (Amount per Serving)

Protein: 4.2 g
Carbs: 8.3 g
Fat: 17.4 g
Sugar: 0.6 g
Calories: 197
Cholesterol: 0 mg

LUNCH RECIPE

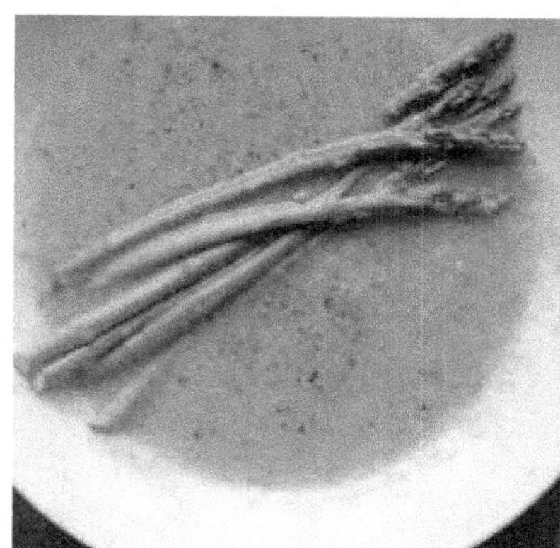

CAULIFLOWER ASPARAGUS SOUP

Serves: 4
Prep Time: 30 minutes

Ingredients

- 20 asparagus spears, chopped
- 4 cups vegetable stock
- ½ cauliflower head, chopped
- 2 garlic cloves, chopped
- 1 tbsp coconut oil
- Pepper
- Salt

Directions

1. Heat coconut oil.
2. Add garlic and sauté until softened.
3. Add cauliflower, vegetable stock, pepper, and salt. Stir well and bring to boil.
4. Simmer for 20 minutes.
5. Add chopped asparagus and cook until softened.
6. Stir well and serve warm.

Nutritional Value (Amount per Serving)

Protein: 3.4 g
Carbs: 8.9 g
Fat: 5.6 g
Sugar: 5.1 g
Calories: 74
Cholesterol: 2 mg

DINNER RECIPE

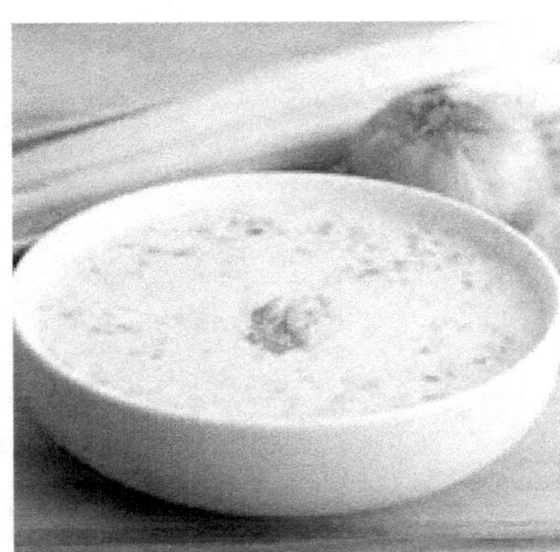

Creamy Celery Soup

Serves: 4
Prep Time: 40 minutes

Ingredients

- 6 cups celery
- ½ tsp dill
- 2 cups water
- 1 cup coconut milk
- 1 onion, chopped
- Pinch of salt

Directions

1. Add all ingredients and stir well.
2. Cover instant pot with lid and select soup setting.
3. Stir well and serve warm.

Nutritional Value (Amount per Serving)

Protein: 2.8 g
Carbs: 10.5 g
Fat: 14.6 g
Sugar: 5.2 g
Calories: 174
Cholesterol: 0 mg

Day 26

Shopping list

- Tofu
- Non-dairy milk
- Onion
- Jalapeno
- Tomatoes
- Cilantro
- Potato
- Tortilla wraps
- Chili powder
- Salt and pepper
- Lemon juice
- Lime juice
- Clove garlic
- Avocado
- Black beans
- Cumin
- Chili powder
- Garlic powder
- Portobello mushroom caps
- Red bell pepper
- Orange bell pepper
- Salt and pepper
- Virgin olive oil
- Spinach
- Potatoes
- Spinach
- Parsley
- Carrots
- Vegetable broth

BREAKFAST RECIPE

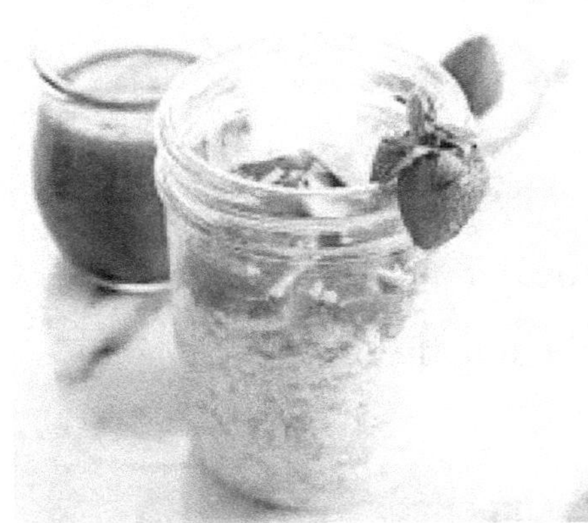

GRAIN-FREE OVERNIGHT OATS

Serves: 1
Prep Time: 10 minutes

Ingredients

- 2/3 cup unsweetened coconut milk
- 2 tsp chia seeds
- 2 tbsp vanilla protein powder
- ½ tbsp coconut flour
- 3 tbsp hemp hearts

Directions

1. Add all ingredients into the glass jar and stir to combine.
2. Close jar with lid and place in refrigerator for overnight.
3. Top with fresh berries and serve.

Nutritional Value (Amount per Serving)

Protein: 27 g
Carbs: 15 g
Fat: 22.5 g
Sugar: 1.5 g
Calories: 378
Cholesterol: 0 mg

LUNCH RECIPE

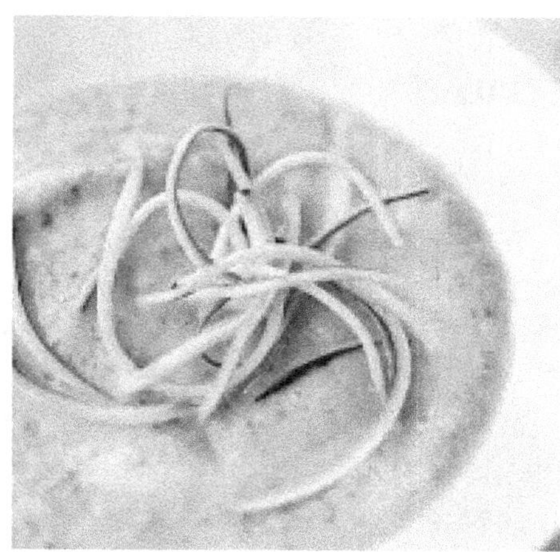

ZUCCHINI SOUP

Serves: 8
Prep Time: 20 minutes

Ingredients

- 2 ½ lbs zucchini, peeled and sliced
- 1/3 cup basil leaves
- 4 cups vegetable stock
- 4 garlic cloves, chopped
- 2 tbsp olive oil
- 1 medium onion, diced
- Pepper
- Salt

Directions

1. Heat olive oil.
2. Add zucchini and onion and sauté until softened. Add garlic and sauté for a minute.
3. Simmer for 15 minutes.
4. Remove from heat. Stir in basil and puree the soup using a blender until smooth and creamy. Season with pepper and salt.
5. Stir well and serve.

Nutritional Value (Amount per Serving)

Protein: 2 g
Carbs: 6.8 g
Fat: 4 g
Sugar: 3.3 g
Calories: 62
Cholesterol: 0 mg

DINNER RECIPE

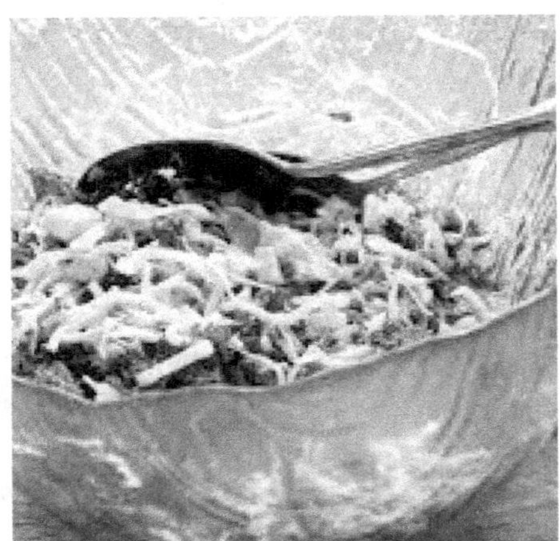

Avocado Almond Cabbage Salad

Serves: 3
Prep Time: 15 minutes

Ingredients

- 3 cups savoy cabbage, shredded
- ½ cup blanched almonds
- 1 avocado, chopped
- ¼ tsp pepper
- ¼ tsp sea salt
- For dressing:

- 1 tsp coconut aminos
- ½ tsp Dijon mustard
- 1 tbsp lemon juice
- 3 tbsp olive oil
- Pepper
- Salt

Directions

1. Mix together all dressing ingredients and set aside.
2. Add all salad ingredients to the large bowl and mix well.
3. Pour dressing over salad and toss well.
4. Serve immediately and enjoy.

Nutritional Value (Amount per Serving)

Protein: 11.6 g
Carbs: 39.8 g
Fat: 14.1 g
Sugar: 9.3 g
Calories: 317
Cholesterol: 0 mg

Day 27

Shopping list

- Tofu
- Non-dairy milk
- Onion
- Jalapeno
- Tomatoes
- Cilantro
- Potato
- Tortilla wraps
- Chili powder
- Salt and pepper
- Lemon juice
- Lime juice
- Clove garlic
- Avocado
- Black beans
- Cumin
- Chili powder
- Garlic powder
- Portobello mushroom caps
- Red bell pepper
- Orange bell pepper
- Salt and pepper
- Virgin olive oil
- Spinach
- Potatoes
- Spinach
- Parsley
- Carrots
- Vegetable broth

BREAKFAST RECIPE

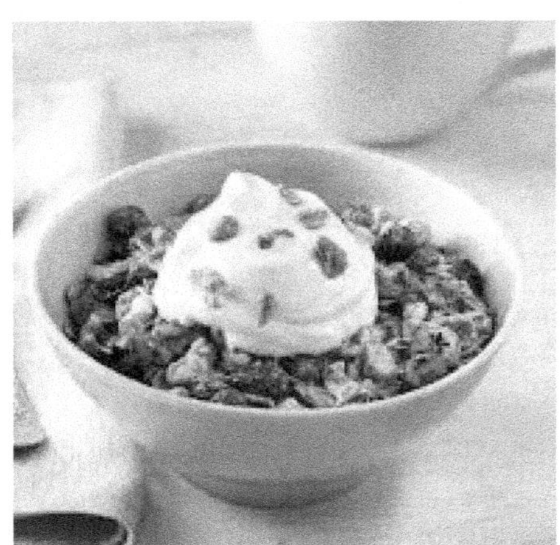

BREAKFAST GRANOLA

Serves: 15
Prep Time: 30 minutes

Ingredients

- 1 tsp ground ginger
- 1 tsp ground cinnamon
- ¼ cups coconut oil, melted
- 1 cup walnuts, chopped
- 2/3 cup pumpkin seeds
- 2/3 cup sunflower seeds
- ½ cup flaxseeds
- 3 cups desiccated coconut

Directions

1. Add all ingredients

2. Spread granola mixture on a baking tray and bake at 350 F/ 180 C for 20 minutes. Turn granola mixture with a spoon after every 3 minutes.

3. Allow to cool completely and serve.

Nutritional Value (Amount per Serving)

Protein: 4.1 g
Carbs: 11.4 g
Fat: 17 g
Sugar: 5.8 g
Calories: 208
Cholesterol: 0 mg

LUNCH RECIPE

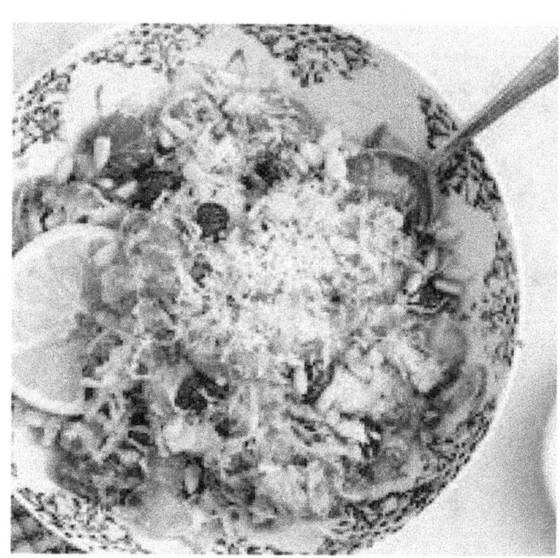

Brussels sprouts Salad

Serves: 6
Prep Time: 20 minutes

Ingredients

- 1 ½ lbs Brussels sprouts, trimmed
- ¼ cup toasted hazelnuts, chopped
- 2 tsp Dijon mustard
- 1 ½ tbsp lemon juice
- 2 tbsp olive oil
- Pepper
- Salt

Directions

1. Whisk together oil, mustard, lemon juice, pepper, and salt.
2. In a large bowl, combine together Brussels sprouts and hazelnuts.
3. Pour dressing over salad and toss well.
4. Serve immediately and enjoy.

Nutritional Value (Amount per Serving)

Protein: 4.4 g
Carbs: 11 g
Fat: 7.1 g
Sugar: 2.7 g
Calories: 111
Cholesterol: 0 mg

DINNER RECIPE

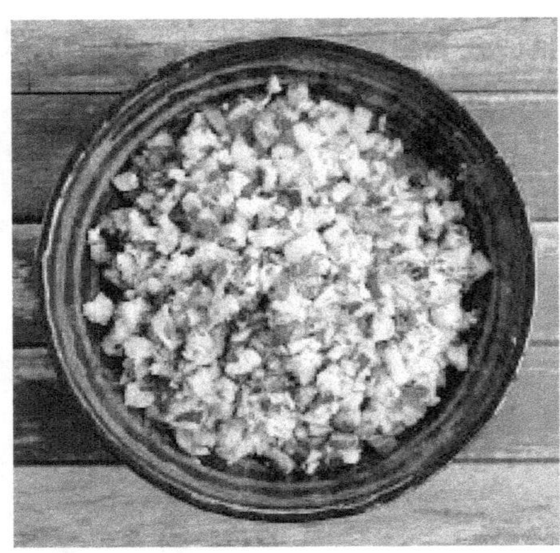

Cauliflower Radish Salad

Serves: 4
Prep Time: 15 minutes

Ingredients

- 12 radishes, trimmed and chopped
- 1 tsp dried dill
- 1 tsp Dijon mustard
- 1 tbsp cider vinegar
- 1 tbsp olive oil
- 1 cup parsley, chopped
- ½ medium cauliflower head, trimmed and chopped
- ½ tsp black pepper
- ¼ tsp sea salt

Directions

1. In a mixing bowl, combine together cauliflower, parsley, and radishes.
2. In a small bowl, whisk together olive oil, dill, mustard, vinegar, pepper, and salt.
3. Pour dressing over salad and toss well.
4. Serve immediately and enjoy.

Nutritional Value (Amount per Serving)

Protein: 2.1 g
Carbs: 5.6 g
Fat: 3.8 g
Sugar: 2.1 g
Calories: 58
Cholesterol: 0 mg

Day 28

Shopping list

- Tofu
- Non-dairy milk
- Onion
- Jalapeno
- Tomatoes
- Cilantro
- Potato
- Tortilla wraps
- Chili powder
- Salt and pepper
- Lemon juice
- Lime juice
- Clove garlic
- Avocado
- Black beans
- Cumin
- Chili powder
- Garlic powder
- Portobello mushroom caps
- Red bell pepper
- Orange bell pepper
- Salt and pepper
- Virgin olive oil
- Spinach
- Potatoes
- Spinach
- Parsley
- Carrots
- Vegetable broth

BREAKFAST RECIPE

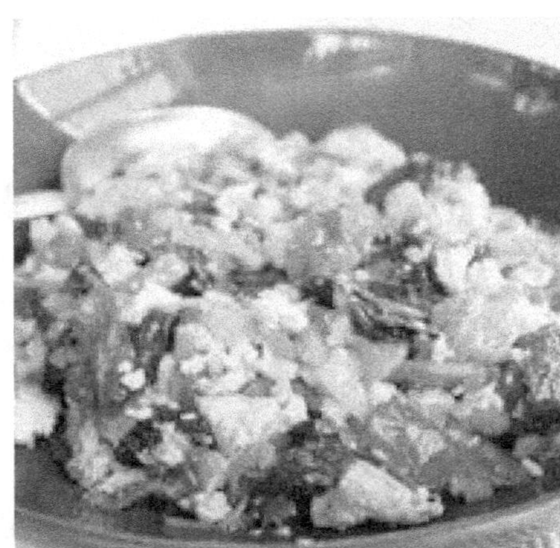

VEGETABLE TOFU SCRAMBLE

Serves: 2
Prep Time: 20 minutes

Ingredients

- 1 block firm tofu, drained and crumbled
- ½ tsp turmeric
- ¼ tsp garlic powder
- 1 cup spinach
- 1 red pepper, chopped
- 10 oz mushrooms, chopped
- ½ onion, chopped
- 1 tbsp olive oil
- Pepper
- Salt

Directions

1. Heat olive oil.
2. Add onion, pepper, and mushrooms and sauté until cooked.
3. Add crumbled tofu, spices, and spinach. Stir well and cook for 3-5 minutes.
4. Serve and enjoy.

Nutritional Value (Amount per Serving)

Protein: 9.6 g
Carbs: 13.7 g
Fat: 9.6 g
Sugar: 7 g
Calories: 159
Cholesterol: 0 mg

LUNCH RECIPE

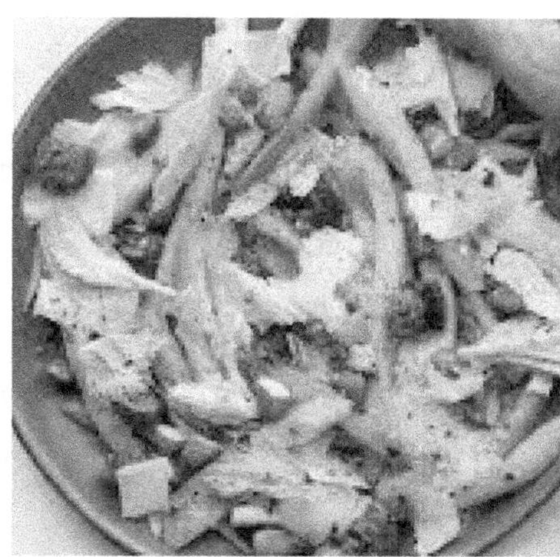

CELERY SALAD

Serves: 6
Prep Time: 10 minutes

Ingredients

- 6 cups celery, sliced
- ¼ tsp celery seed
- 1 tbsp lemon juice
- 2 tsp lemon zest, grated
- 1 tbsp parsley, chopped
- 1 tbsp olive oil
- Sea salt

Directions

1. Add all ingredients
2. Serve immediately and enjoy.

Nutritional Value (Amount per Serving)

Protein: 0.8 g
Carbs: 3.3 g
Fat: 2.5 g
Sugar: 1.5 g
Calories: 38
Cholesterol: 0 mg

DINNER RECIPE

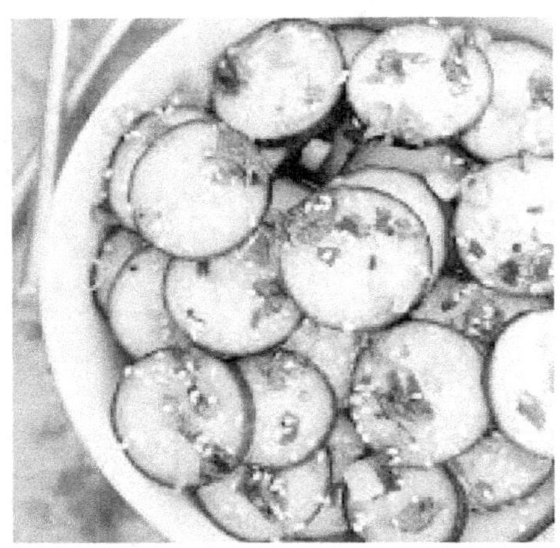

Asian Cucumber Salad

Serves: 6
Prep Time: 10 minutes

Ingredients

- 4 cups cucumbers, sliced
- ¼ tsp red pepper flakes
- ½ tsp sesame oil
- 1 tsp sesame seeds
- ¼ cup rice wine vinegar
- ¼ cup red pepper, diced
- ¼ cup onion, sliced
- ½ tsp sea salt

Directions

1. Add all ingredients and toss well.
2. Serve immediately and enjoy.

Nutritional Value (Amount per Serving)

Protein: 0.7 g
Carbs: 3.5 g
Fat: 0.7 g
Sugar: 1.6 g
Calories: 27
Cholesterol: 0 mg

Day 29

Shopping list

- Tofu
- Non-dairy milk
- Onion
- Jalapeno
- Tomatoes
- Cilantro
- Potato
- Tortilla wraps
- Chili powder
- Salt and pepper
- Lemon juice
- Lime juice
- Clove garlic
- Avocado
- Black beans
- Cumin
- Chili powder
- Garlic powder
- Portobello mushroom caps
- Red bell pepper
- Orange bell pepper
- Salt and pepper
- Virgin olive oil
- Spinach
- Potatoes
- Spinach
- Parsley
- Carrots
- Vegetable broth

BREAKFAST RECIPE

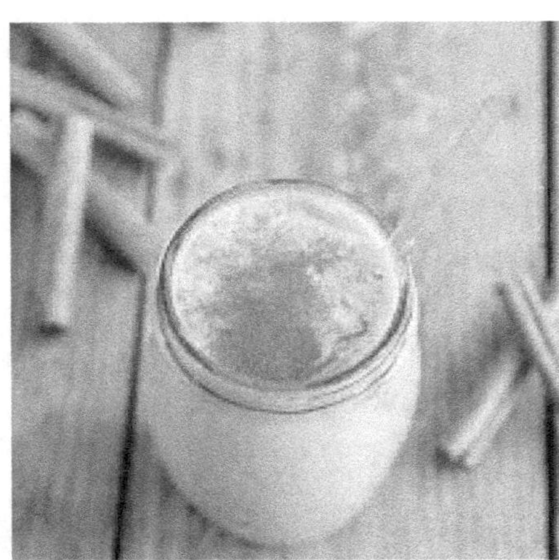

CHIA CINNAMON SMOOTHIE

Serves: 1
Prep Time: 5 minutes

Ingredients

- 2 scoops vanilla protein powder
- 1 tbsp chia seeds
- ½ tsp cinnamon
- 1 tbsp coconut oil
- ½ cup water
- ½ cup unsweetened coconut milk

Directions

1. Blend until smooth and creamy.
2. Serve immediately and enjoy.

Nutritional Value (Amount per Serving)

Protein: 31.6 g
Carbs: 13.4 g
Fat: 23.9 g
Sugar: 0 g
Calories: 397
Cholesterol: 0 mg

LUNCH RECIPE

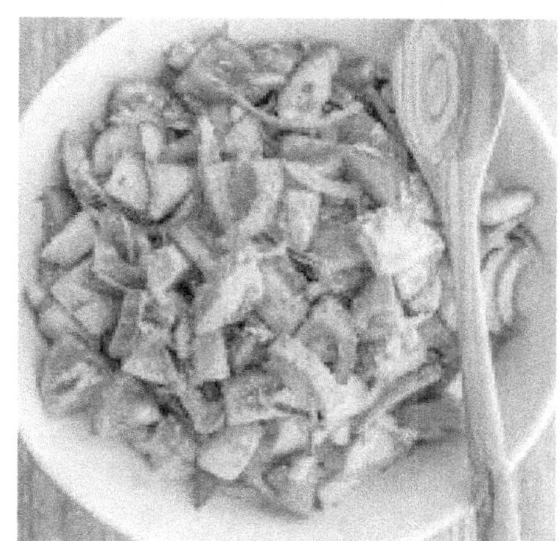

Tomato Avocado Cucumber Salad

Serves: 4
Prep Time: 10 minutes

Ingredients

- 1 cucumber, sliced
- 2 avocados, chopped
- ½ onion, sliced
- 2 tomatoes, chopped
- 1 bell pepper, chopped
- For dressing:
- 2 tbsp cilantro
- ¼ tsp garlic powder
- 2 tbsp olive oil
- 1 tbsp lemon juice
- ½ tsp black pepper
- ½ tsp salt

Directions

1. Mix together all dressing ingredients and set aside.
2. Add all salad ingredients into the large mixing bowl and mix well.
3. Pour dressing over salad and toss well.
4. Serve immediately and enjoy.

Nutritional Value (Amount per Serving)

Protein: 2.1 g
Carbs: 10.6 g
Fat: 9.8 g
Sugar: 5.1 g
Calories: 130
Cholesterol: 0 mg

DINNER RECIPE

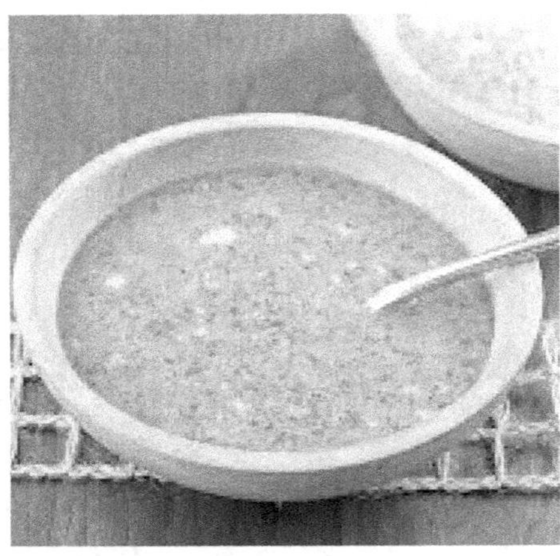

Avocado Broccoli Soup

Serves: 4
Prep Time: 25 minutes

Ingredients

- 2 cups broccoli florets, chopped
- 5 cups vegetable broth
- 2 avocados, chopped
- Pepper
- Salt

Directions

1. Cook broccoli. Drain well.
2. Add broccoli, vegetable broth, avocados, pepper, and salt to the blender and blend until smooth.
3. Stir well and serve warm.

Nutritional Value (Amount per Serving)

Protein: 9.2 g
Carbs: 12.8 g
Fat: 21.5 g
Sugar: 2.1 g
Calories: 269
Cholesterol: 0 mg

Day 30

Shopping list

- Tofu
- Non-dairy milk
- Onion
- Jalapeno
- Tomatoes
- Cilantro
- Potato
- Tortilla wraps
- Chili powder
- Salt and pepper
- Lemon juice
- Lime juice
- Clove garlic
- Avocado
- Black beans
- Cumin
- Chili powder
- Garlic powder
- Portobello mushroom caps
- Red bell pepper
- Orange bell pepper
- Salt and pepper
- Virgin olive oil
- Spinach
- Potatoes
- Spinach
- Parsley
- Carrots
- Vegetable broth

BREAKFAST RECIPE

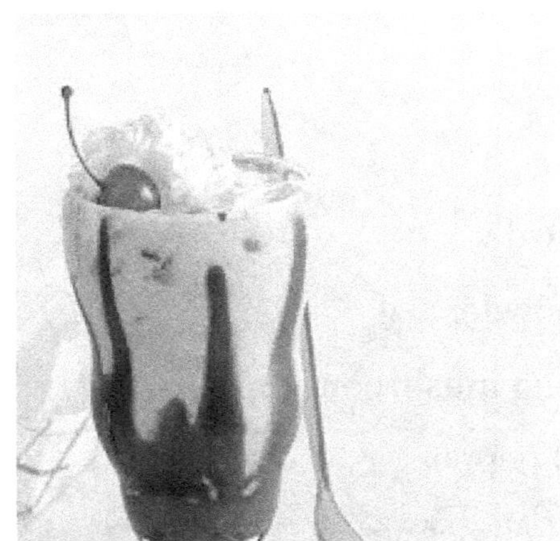

CHOCOLATE STRAWBERRY MILKSHAKE

Serves: 2
Prep Time: 5 minutes

Ingredients

- 1 cup ice cubes
- ¼ cup unsweetened cocoa powder
- 2 scoops vegan protein powder
- 1 cup strawberries
- 2 cups unsweetened coconut milk

Directions

1. Add all ingredients and blend until smooth and creamy.
2. Serve immediately and enjoy.

Nutritional Value (Amount per Serving)

Protein: 27.7 g
Carbs: 15 g
Fat: 5.7 g
Sugar: 6.8 g
Calories: 221
Cholesterol: 0 mg

LUNCH RECIPE

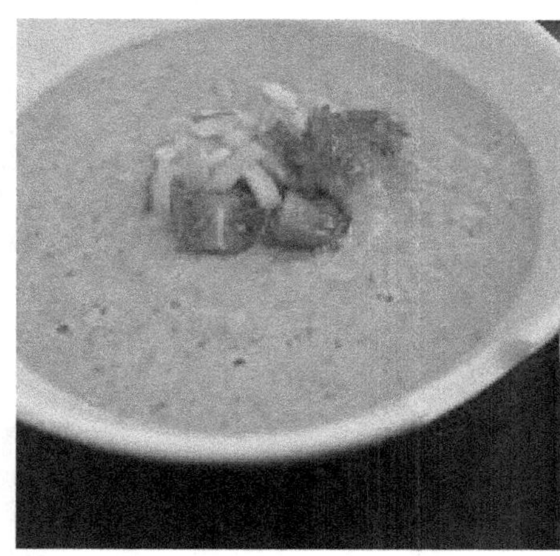

Avocado Cucumber Soup

Serves: 3
Prep Time: 40 minutes

Ingredients

- 1 large cucumber, peeled and sliced
- ¾ cup water
- ¼ cup lemon juice
- 2 garlic cloves
- 6 green onion
- 2 avocados, pitted
- ½ tsp black pepper
- ½ tsp pink salt

Directions

1. Add all ingredients into the blender and blend until smooth and creamy.
2. Place in refrigerator for 30 minutes.
3. Stir well and serve chilled.

Nutritional Value (Amount per Serving)

Protein: 2.2 g
Carbs: 9.2 g
Fat: 3.7 g
Sugar: 2.8 g
Calories: 73
Cholesterol: 0 mg

DINNER RECIPE

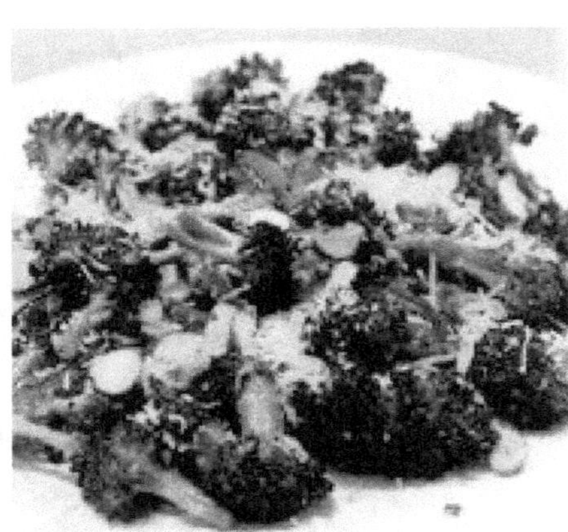

Roasted Almond Broccoli

Serves: 4
Prep Time: 25 minutes

Ingredients

- 1 1/2 lbs broccoli florets
- 3 tbsp olive oil
- 1 tbsp fresh lemon juice
- 3 tbsp slivered almonds, toasted
- 2 garlic cloves, sliced
- 1/4 tsp pepper
- 1/4 tsp salt

Directions

1. The oven to be preheated to 425 F/ 218 C.
2. Spray baking dish with cooking spray.
3. Add broccoli, pepper, salt, garlic, and oil in large bowl and toss well.
4. Spread broccoli on the prepared baking dish and roast in preheated oven for 20 minutes.
5. Add lemon juice and almonds over broccoli and toss well.
6. Serve and enjoy.

Nutritional Value (Amount per Serving)

Protein: 5.8 g
Carbs: 12.9 g
Fat: 13.3 g
Sugar: 3.2 g
Calories: 177
Cholesterol: 0 mg

CHAPTER 6:

Maintaining a progress journal

One thing that I have heard so many people worry and stress about when beginning to adopt a vegan diet is that they will miss the meat, or they're worried about how to get the protein and iron. I've even had so many friends think they couldn't do it because they would miss meat so much and they were scared they wouldn't be able to keep it up over time. So whether you're just becoming a vegan now or you already are one, we're going to tell you how to start on this diet and how to stay on this diet. The one thing I recommend the most is if you're really worried about cutting meat from your diet, go slow. You can be at a dinner with a few friends and they want to share an appetizer and you think one won't hurt, or they want to drink so you figure one drink won't have too many carbs or something along those lines. A quick tip though; a lot of drinks do have carbs and on a ketogenic diet, it is really not recommended because you'll bust straight through your numbers. Some people even give in to the peer pressure because their friends get upset that someone is not eating like the rest of them. Also, if it helps, there are so many yummy alternatives to meat and you can find them at just about any supermarket which should make the switch even easier. Another thing to remind people is that once you begin adjusting to this diet, you will probably begin to crave meat less and less. Many people have said that they have been vegan for most of their lives and don't miss meat at all. Others say they feel bad for the meat eaters who are missing out on what vegetarians and vegans enjoy every day, from the great health benefits of the food to the wonderful flavors of the new foods in their diet.

A good tip to start out is do not go cold turkey. No pun intended. When you go cold turkey without adequate preparation, you tend to be more likely to go back to eating meat and your old diet. Then you feel guilty and it can be a bad cycle. Removing it slowly over time is the best way to go about this because you're familiarizing your body to the new food and letting go of the old. Over time, you'll notice that you're craving meat less and the switch will become easier. A good example to go with is let's say you're trying to cut sweets out of your diet. So you remove anything with sugar in your house. Then you start to eat healthy for maybe a few hours or a day and you begin to get cravings. The problem with many people is that they get so hungry because they don't have the proper research about what to eat, and then they end up going on a binge or running out to the nearest place with cookies or they stay home, and binge eat. Now, you might think binging on healthy food is better but it's not. Binge eating is never healthy and can lead to eating disorders which are a bad thing.

Later, you feel guilty and ashamed which only hurts you and your progress as well as your emotional being. If you slip up, remember you are human. It can happen to anyone and there is no reason to feel guilty or ashamed. Slip-ups happen. It is also important to note that slip-ups will probably happen in the first couple of days and if they do, it's alright. The important thing is that you're trying to better yourself and that you want to change. This is a good thing. Reminding yourself of that will help guide you because you will be able to understand that the effort you're putting forth is something to be proud of and one day you won't slip up at all.

You should also begin adding to your diet before taking things away. Familiarize yourself with how you prepare your new food, how it's stored, and the uses they have. With studying, you will see that many of your items can be used as multipurpose items. Olive oil is great for your skin and hair just as one example of how it can be used in a different way. You should start adding more vegan staples but keep in mind that you're both a vegan and ketogenic, not just one or the other. This means that there are certain things that ketogenic eat that vegans don't; like fish or meat for ketogenic; for vegans, most eat beans or potatoes and starchy foods but ketogenic usually avoid them because of the high carb content. So when adding things to your diet, keep in mind what you need to avoid and what will bring the most benefits to your new lifestyle.

Make sure you stay informed. You need to make sure you've got good information going into this because that will help you know what you can and can't eat, or wear or use on your body. Also, stay up to date on science and studies. People are still researching these diets and lifestyles to give people the correct information. If you stay up to date, you'll be able to see the new information too.

If you feel like you can't do it, remind yourself why you decided to do this in the first place. Remind yourself of the facts. Watch videos online or read studies. They say its harder to slip when you see the facts presented to you and you're watching the consequences of eating meat.

Offer to make dinner for your friends or ask if you can make some vegan dishes to a dinner or party. More often than not, you will see that they're really interested in what you have to say and that they will love how amazing your food tastes. They may even opt to go vegan themselves! A perfect example is let's say all your meat-eater friends are having a dinner party and want you to bring a dessert. Okay, easy peasy. Make them some vegan keto zucchini brownies, or some vegan keto cupcakes and watch them fall in love. I bet you won't even be able to tell that there are healthy vegetables in there and your friends will fall in love.

Make your lifestyle the new norm. Everyone thinks that meat-eating is the norm; switch what it means. Now, this doesn't mean getting in people's faces and being rude or abrupt. Be kind and polite. Be happy in the knowledge that you're making a difference and try to feel compassionate to people no matter what choices they make. If you are content with who you are, it is more likely that people will be open to talking to you about this. They could even begin questioning their own choices. But by simply being an awesome and secure person who's happy in their choices, you'll probably begin to see that your friends want to come to you because they see you so happy and want to know what your secret is.

Finding new items and recipes can be a fun and exciting adventure and a great way to keep yourself on track. We can always learn new things and for a lot of people, going on little adventures can be a lot of fun. Get out and about and see what vegan things you can find around you.

Find inspiration. There are so many celebrities that have taken up the cause and so many other people as well. Doctors, lawyers, teachers; there are so many people now that have joined the vegan move. There are also many organizations that have taken up the movement as well. Be careful with these organizations though and make sure they are on the up and up. Studies have shown that some organizations kill more animals than they save. Or some don't follow the ideas you have for yourself. You need to make sure that you find inspiration that is going to help you. Thanks to social media, you can even be connected to hundreds of thousands of people that have the same lifestyle and desires to help animals as you do. You can ask questions and learn everything you can about the vegan lifestyle. As with anything on social media though, you need to be careful as there are dangers beyond bad advice as some people simply can't be trusted so you'll need to be careful that you don't get hurt.

Grow your own food. This one not everyone can do. But if you can, grow your own food. You could grow the food you eat and earn a deeper appreciation for your food and what's going in your body.

You'll be able to see the work and effort it takes to provide yourself sustenance and you might even help other people try new things because the tastes are different. You can grow anything from vegetables to spices. The really cool thing though is if there's something you want to eat but can't find it anywhere, you can grow it yourself. Now, obviously, if you have to grow it, you won't get it when you want it because it would take weeks or months before it would be ready to eat. However, you will be able to have access to it which is a pretty cool thing to think about. If your garden got big enough, you could share with your finds and family and maybe they would be interested in eating healthier foods for themselves and their family because of your example.

Another surprising thing in this digital age is that you can have groceries delivered to you, even fresh ones in certain cases. This might help people who don't have vegan options near them. It will be easier for you to have it delivered especially if you live far away from the city or you're far from a place that actually carries what you need. Online shopping can also be a great way to try some new snacks as long as you're making sure it's not junk food or overly processed stuff that is going to make you gain a lot of weight. Look for options you know are good.

Remember, this is a journey. If you slip up, forgive and motivate yourself to do better so it won't happen again. If you're tired of the current options you're eating, find/keep trying new recipes and foods that you love. Keep looking around and exploring so that your knowledge keeps expanding. This can be a really fun way to make yourself happy and healthy and make sure that you accomplish the goals that you want to reach for yourself.

CONCLUSION

Plant-based diet is not as complicated as you think it is and most of the ingredients are easy to get, in fact, you might even plant them at your backyard! Unlike the regular diet ingredients, in a situation where you have to find a specific animal parts, some places may run out of them and you might crave for the dish for God knows how long until the parts are available again. Meanwhile, plant-based ingredients are abundant and could be find at your nearest stores or street vendors, at a much lower cost too!

Making a decision to structure how your plant-based diet is going to look is the first step, and it is going to help you transition from your current diet outlook. This is something that is really personal and varies from one person to the other. While some people decide that they will not tolerate any animal products at all, some make do with tiny bits of dairy or meat occasionally. It is really up to you to decide what and how you want your plant-based diet to look like. The most important thing is that whole plant-based foods have to make a great majority of your diet.

I may not be able to ask people to start eating plant-based foods, but it's good enough to make them aware of the nutrition that they consumed daily in their food plan. Furthermore, I cannot change their mind about how easy it is to cook plant-based meals, but at least they could try these recipes at home and that would make them start pondering on the coolness of practicing a plant-based diet one day.

PLANT-BASED KETO COOKBOOK